Multilingual Practices and Monolingual Mindsets

Focusing on health care interpreting in Australia, this book examines the under-recognition of interpreting from a critical sociolinguistic perspective encompassing language, race and class.

Interpreters play an important role in promoting diversity and inclusion but why is interpreting not properly recognised? Cho grapples with this question by focusing readers' attention to developments in interpreting following increased migration in an English-monolingual Australia, a context in which other languages and speakers have been historically under-valued. Through compelling analysis and the voices of health care interpreters in Australia, this groundbreaking book explores how issues with interpreting are fundamentally issues of justice that affect minority languages and their speakers. Covering diverse professional and social spaces of interpreting, the book discovers linguistic, racial and class hierarchies embedded in English monolingualism and their impact on multilingual practices and populations. From both historical and contemporary perspectives, the book critically investigates monolingual practices from the past and tensions between enduring monolingual ideologies and multilingual realities, suggesting specific ways to overcome monolingual mindsets to make societies more inclusive.

This volume will be of interest to students and scholars in interpreting studies, health communication, intercultural communication and sociolinguistics.

Jinhyun Cho is a senior lecturer in the Department of Linguistics at Macquarie University. Her research cuts across translation/interpreting and sociolinguistics, with a focus on language ideologies, language policies and intercultural communication. With a novel approach, which sees interpreting as social activities infused with power, her research has captured the dynamics of cultural, linguistic, and ethnic power relations in diverse sociolinguistic contexts.

Routledge Advances in Translation and Interpreting Studies

The Translator's Visibility
New Debates and Epistemologies
Edited by Larisa Cercel and Alice Leal

Translation on Display
Multilingual Texts in Multimodal Museum Space
Min-Hsiu Liao

Translation, Pornography, Performativity
Experimenting with That Dangerous Supplement
Douglas Robinson and Xiaorui Sun

Chinese Political Discourse in Translation
A Corpus-based Critical Discourse Analysis
Lijuan Du

Retour Interpreting
The Art of Interpreting into B
Edited by Riccardo Moratto and Irene A. Zhang

Humanizing Critical Journalistic Translation Studies
Insights from the Chinese Context
Ali Jalalian Daghigh and Pei Soo Ang

Multilingual Practices and Monolingual Mindsets
Critical Sociolinguistic Perspectives on Health Care Interpreting
Jinhyun Cho

For more information about this series, please visit: www.routledge.com/Routledge-Advances-in-Translation-and-Interpreting-Studies/book-series/RTS

Multilingual Practices and Monolingual Mindsets

Critical Sociolinguistic Perspectives on Health Care Interpreting

Jinhyun Cho

Routledge
Taylor & Francis Group
NEW YORK AND LONDON

First published 2025
by Routledge
605 Third Avenue, New York, NY 10158

and by Routledge
4 Park Square, Milton Park, Abingdon, Oxon, OX14 4RN

Routledge is an imprint of the Taylor & Francis Group, an informa business

ISBN: 9781032614847 (hbk)
ISBN: 9781032614878 (pbk)
ISBN: 9781032614854 (ebk)

DOI: 10.4324/9781032614854

Typeset in Sabon
by Newgen Publishing UK

To Peter, Justin and Daniel

Contents

Acknowledgement

Writing is an act of questioning. I wanted to ask questions about people who make significant contributions to social inclusion yet remain excluded from social attention: interpreters. This book explores how and why interpreters remain invisible and under-appreciated in Australian society characterised by linguistic, racial and class hierarchies. By exposing social inequalities embedded in interpreting, I wanted to draw attention to the nature of power which is sustained through the normalisation of the hierarchies in places in which it is least visible.

No research is standalone, and this book owes much to the work of the researchers who paid attention to the first health care interpreters in Australia in the 1970s. Without those records, it would have been impossible to write this book. I would also like to extend deepest gratitude to the interpreters who participated in the research. Some participants did not want to receive a reward for their research participation, asking me to use the funds to help people in need. While I could not do that due to the research funding regulations, I very much appreciate their humanism and commitment to helping the vulnerable.

This research was funded by the Macquarie University Research Acceleration Scheme, and I am grateful to the University for enabling the study. Without its generous support, writing this book would have been impossible.

Finally, I would like to acknowledge my family, who have been my biggest supporters throughout my career journeys. The occasional, inevitable agony in the process of writing books was alleviated by the daily laughs and experiences we shared as a family, for which I am truly grateful.

This book is dedicated to all interpreters from the past and in the present.

1 Questioning interpreting in society

1.1 A tale of two interpreters

Here are stories of two interpreters:

> One was born in Korea and became interested in interpreting, specifically interpreting between English and Korean. As a young girl, she found people speaking English fluently very cool and thought that English-Korean interpreters appearing on television were the coolest of them all. To become an interpreter specialising in English, she dedicated herself to intensive English language learning for many years and finally got into a prestigious interpreting school in Korea. Upon graduation, she landed a job at a large multinational, where she was responsible for global communication through translation and interpreting. Wherever she goes, she is envied by people for her fluency in English. When people find out that she is an English-Korean interpreter working for a global company, they immediately show interest and ask for tips on how to become fluent in English. Although she finds it stressful to live up to external expectations of her language skills, being an interpreter also makes her feel proud due to the social recognition of the profession.
>
> The other interpreter was born in Korea too, yet migrated to Australia as a young girl with her family. She picked up English quickly and acted as a child interpreter for her parents who had trouble managing daily life due to their limited English language proficiency. From this experience, she learned how important a role interpreting plays for migrants unable to speak English well and decided to become an interpreter to help people in need. After taking a relevant course at a vocational school, she passed an interpreting exam and has worked as a health care interpreter ever since. When people find out she is an interpreter, few show much interest. The general perception is that interpreting is just a job, rather than a genuine profession. People including health care providers tend to think that anyone who knows more than one

DOI: 10.4324/9781032614854-1

language can interpret. Although the interpreter finds it rewarding to help people in need, being an interpreter also makes her feel ambivalent about her professional identity.

The stories are based on the real experiences of over 150 interpreters including 67 health care interpreters in Australia whose stories serve as a basis for this book. Over the past decade, I have had conversations with interpreters from Australia and Korea to explore various sociolinguistic dimensions of interpreting. As our conversations continued, the contrasts in terms of the societal recognition of interpreting between the two countries became all too clear.[1]

I started asking why it is that interpreting is highly regarded in some countries, while the same profession is under-appreciated in others. In migrant-receiving countries such as Australia, community (or 'public service') interpreters serving minority groups make invaluable contributions to helping the marginalised to access key services (e.g., education, hospital, law and welfare). Without interpreters, linguistic minorities will be denied resources critical for leading the lives they deserve as human beings. Interpreting, therefore, has direct implications on access equity for vulnerable groups. Despite its centrality to social inclusion, why is interpreting under-appreciated? How does the under-recognition of interpreting impact the ways interpreters work and how does it relate to broader social attitudes to other languages and speakers?

This book was inspired by these initial questions. In trying to address them, there are three important points of departure relating to language, race and class in interpreting.

First, while bilingualism is highly valued in many countries such as Korea, monolingualism embedded in English is a societal norm in Australia. Many people in Korea, for example, make a huge amount of investment to acquire proficiency in foreign languages, particularly in English, which represents valuable capital in both material and symbolic terms (Cho, 2017). People fluent in English such as interpreters are, therefore, highly respected for their language proficiency. Admiration of English and interpreters can also be found in China in which some interpreters even enjoy celebrity status (Du & Wang, 2021).

In contrast, languages other than English are hardly valued in Australia. With nearly 30 per cent of the population born overseas and over 300 languages spoken across the country, Australia is not only multicultural but also multilingual. Languages other than English are, however, literally invisible, with English governing all aspects of life in Australia. The domination of English is so strong that the country is referred to as a "monolingual multicultural society" (Adoniou, 2018, p. 274). The under-appreciation of interpreting exemplified in the story of the second interpreter needs to be understood within this societal context of English monolingualism.

Second, the ethnic profiles of interpreters show a marked difference between the two countries. In Korea, interpreters are generally local people both born and brought up there. All interpreter-participants from Korea for the research I have conducted, for example, were Korean nationals. While migrant-background interpreters serving ethnic communities are increasing in the country in the context of increasing inbound migration (Lee et al., 2016), the profession of interpreting has been traditionally occupied by locals. And they generally work in high-profile areas including foreign affairs and multinational business, serving privileged 'expats' rather than 'foreigners'.

As a major migrant-receiving country, Australia, however, features a very different picture in terms of interpreters' ethnic profiles. Interpreters are predominantly migrants speaking their ethnic language as their first language, while speaking English with an accent (Cho, 2021a). Furthermore, community interpreting designed to address the day-to-day needs of migrants from non-English-speaking backgrounds (hereafter 'NESB') has been traditionally dominant in Australia. As such, interpreting there has been strongly associated with foreign status (see Chapter 3 for further details).

Relatedly and finally, there is a notable difference in terms of class. For interpreters in Korea, being a Korean national comes with power and privilege typically out of reach of most migrants. Furthermore, the social recognition of interpreting in sought-after languages such as English endows interpreters with respectable social status in which they are seen as glamorous elite bilinguals (Cho, 2017). Serving powerful figures (e.g., high-ranking businessmen, government officials and international politicians) also helps elevate interpreters' status. This is, however, hardly the case with interpreters in Australia, most of whom are migrants serving migrants. As the interpreter's status and prestige often depend on the person whom they serve, community interpreting tends to suffer a lack of social recognition (see Gentile, 2016).

Interpreting has been traditionally examined as an activity occurring within a communication setting, yet if situated within a broader sociolinguistic context, interpreting represents a site of linguistic, racial and class hierarchies. Focusing on health care interpreting in Australia, this book examines the ties between the under-appreciation of interpreting and monolingualism characterised by linguistic, racial and class hierarchies. From both historical and contemporary perspectives, it examines the processes by which interpreting has suffered from a lack of legitimacy and how its under-recognition has become normalised within English-monolingual Australia.

Drawing on the real stories of 67 health care interpreters in Australia, the book adopts a critical sociolinguistic perspective to provide in-depth and comprehensive accounts of the struggles of the dominated against the dominant. Importantly, it seeks ways to make interpreting visible to promote social inclusion of minority populations.

1.2 Social approaches to interpreting

Following the social turn of interpreting in the late 20th century, interpreting scholars have increasingly adopted sociological approaches to interpreting to illuminate the relevance of social factors to acts of interpreting. By conceptualising interpreting as a socially situated activity (Inghilleri, 2003, 2005) as opposed to the traditional conduit model of interpreting, the sociology of interpreting has focused on society in interpreting as well as interpreting in society. This approach has problematised the notion of interpreters' invisibility, which refers to the dominant belief that "interpreters are not considered to be parties to the conversation, but rather they are seen as language-switching operators in line with the conduit model of communication" (Angelelli, 2004b, p. 7). Furthermore, this line of inquiry has paid attention to interpreters, a previously neglected area due to the exclusive focus on interpreting, by exploring interpreters' identity and agency (e.g., Bahadir, 2017; Baker, 2009; Halley, 2019).

Among others, Bourdieu has been particularly influential in the shift to sociologically informed approaches to the study of interpreting. Moving away from the dominant textual approaches, scholars have applied various Bourdieusian theories, primarily field, capital and habitus, to analyse the interactions between agency and structure in interpreting.

To begin with, field represents a site of contestation in which individuals are engaged in a social game to secure valued capitals (Bourdieu, 1990). As a relatively autonomous area of social life, field represents both a site of forces and a site of struggles, with each having its own rules and sense of the game. If applied to interpreting, the field represents a space which helps to locate interpreting within broader social structures and institutions, through which to analyse how interpreters navigate and negotiate their roles within different social, cultural and political contexts (see Inghilleri, 2005). By examining the cultural, historical, and political specificity of interpreting practices, the field highlights how interpreting is influenced by the specific contexts in which it occurs, including the historical development of the profession and the cultural norms that shape it. This approach has highlighted interpreters as social agents and institutions in which they engage as a microcosm of a wider social field, illustrating how interpreting is constituted in social practices, rather than individual activities separated from the social field (see Giustini, 2016).

Field also represents a site of struggle for interpreters. As a space in which multiple fields intersect, interpreting is occupied by well-established professions (e.g., law and medicine). Agents engaged in these fields possess significant forms of capital recognised by and tied to the objective structure (Colley & Guéry, 2015; Mason & Ren, 2012). Bourdieu defines four forms of capitals – economic, cultural, social and symbolic (Bourdieu, 1986). Economic capital refers to tangible assets (e.g., money and property), while cultural capital tends to be intangible with knowledge, education and skills serving as key examples. Social capital means one's networks including friends, support groups or membership of influential groups. Finally, symbolic capital refers to honour, prestige or forms of legitimation derived from the recognition by others. For symbolic capital to take forms, there needs to be "social consensus about "the value of value"" (Valero Garcés & Gauthier Blasi, 2010, p.4, emphasis in original).

Technically speaking, language skills of interpreters take on rarity value for fluency in multiple languages to the point of interpreting is scarce. Depending on social contexts and type of interpreting, however, the amount of capital generated from interpreting significantly differs. Whereas conference interpreters tend to enjoy economic and symbolic capital in societies having positive attitudes to language, particularly English (see Cho, 2017; Du & Wang, 2021; Giustini, 2022), interpreters working in migrant-receiving countries tend to suffer from a lack of capital. Taking some examples, interpreters working for Syrian refugees in Turkey are underpaid and under-recognised, with their language hardly serving as capital (Ulaş & Gündüz, 2020). The same goes in Australia, where interpreters have struggled due to the low rate of pay and a lack of clear professional identity (Darwish, 2005).

In contrast, established professionals working with interpreters enjoy authority and status endowed by capital tied to social structure, which, in turn, allows these professionals to regenerate and strengthen their positions as legitimate and powerful. In community interpreting, the game is, therefore, not entirely their own, but interpreters are always "*involved in someone else's game* as well as playing their own" (Colley & Guéry, 2015, p. 118, emphasis in original).

Working on the "the 'home terrain' of other more established professions" (Colley & Guéry, 2015, p. 115, emphasis in original), interpreters tend to experience tensions between institutional expectations of interpreting and their own agency (e.g., Ayan, 2020; Cho, 2021b; Tekgül, 2020). The ambivalent positions of interpreters within power structures influence the choices interpreters make over the course of interpreting, and this is well exemplified by the concept of habitus.

Simeoni (1998), who first introduced habitus to translation, defines habitus for translators as the "internalized position of the translator in his field of practice" (p. 12), in which conformity, secondariness and subservience generally serve as a pivot around which translatorial behaviours revolve. Defining translators' habitus as a "locus of tension" (p. 21), Simeoni focuses on the power-laden professional field in which translation takes place to understand the internalised state of the norms which govern translators and translation.

Tensions are not specific to translation but commonly arise in interpreting too. Focusing on monolingualism in legal institutions, Inghilleri (2003) reveals that conflicts in terms of how interpreting should be done often arise due to different perceptions of language between institutions and interpreters. Interpreters understand that what counts as a legitimate meaning often goes beyond surface-level translations. By contrast, legal institutions tend to see interpreting as a word-to-word exercise in which every single word has a matching equivalence and require interpreters to interpret at a word level. Relatedly, interpreters are expected to be invisible, which, in turn, renders interpreters' abilities to make professional judgements and suggestions irrelevant. Under such circumstances, interpreters tend to be seen as machines through which messages are delivered transparently and faithfully, i.e., word-to-word. Habitus is, however, not always conformist yet may also be liberating, albeit momentarily, when interpreters upset the established norm by performing the unexpected such as making cultural and linguistic advice (Inghilleri, 2005). In sum, interpreters' habitus is not fixed yet fluid with the potential of being liberatory within the transient nature of interpreting.

Overall, the extant research indicates that despite the important social contributions made by community interpreting, interpreting is generally under-recognised and low in status (see Angelelli, 2004a; de Pedro Ricoy, 2010; Gentile, 2016; Hale, 2007). Acknowledging the need to enhance the professional status of community interpreting, scholars have suggested systematic training of interpreters, enhanced quality assurance and the professionalisation of community interpreting through the establishment of a central credentialising system (e.g., Dam, 2017; D'Hayer, 2012; Hlavac, 2015; Mikkelson, 1996).

At the same time, however, the question of *why* community interpreting is under-appreciated in relation to societal attitudes to other languages and speakers has hardly been explored. The ties between interpreting and local sociolinguistic conditions are aptly described by Roy and Metzger (2014) who pioneered the sociolinguistics of interpreting:

> ... not only is the sociolinguistic context a relevant aspect of interpretation as a profession, but also the larger sociolinguistic context in which interpreters work. Each interpreted interaction undertaken by a professional interpreter is situated within communities that harbor

> their own unique multilingual, bilingual, and language contact phenomenon; within a setting that represents a snapshot of what may be a long history of language policies and planning; and in a social environment beset with language attitudes about one or both of the languages involved.
>
> (p. 158)

The sociolinguistics of interpreting pays specific attention to local sociolinguistic situations, putting language at the centre of the inquiry into the connections between interpreting and society. It posits that social attitudes to interpreting are inseparable from local sociolinguistic dynamics, which shows interpreting as a unique lens through which to examine linguistic relations embedded in historical and contemporary social contexts.

Sociolinguistic approaches to interpreting have been increasingly adopted by interpreting scholars, yet research has primarily focused on analysing linguistic interactions within interpreter-mediated communication settings based on conversational, interactional and discourse analysis (e.g., Angelelli, 2004b; Aranguri et al., 2006; Diriker, 2003; Wadensjö, 2014). To the best of my knowledge, there is hardly any research which examines the relations between societal monolingualism and public perception of interpreting. It is important to note that in any society, there is a dominant language versus dominated languages, and, by extension, a dominant group speaking the language of power versus dominated groups speaking other undervalued languages (Bourdieu, 1993; see also Section 2.2). In the case of Australia, the country is characterised by its century-old "monolingual mindset" (Clyne, 2005) which sees everything in terms of English. Relatedly, Anglo privilege and the persistent ideology of Australia as a white country have been strongly embedded in Australian consciousness (Piller et al., 2023; see Chapter 3 for details).

In this context of English monolingualism embedded in 'us' and 'them', interpreters predominantly come from the dominated who are linguistic, racial and class others. In the existing scholarship, including both sociology and sociolinguistics of interpreting, interpreters are generally seen as professionals involved in interpreting processes. While communication mediation is a core professional tenet of interpreters, it is worth questioning whether interpreters are immune to entrenched monolingual biases against other languages and speakers. Shifting the focus from interpreters as professionals involved in interpreting processes to interpreters as minorities subject to linguistic, racial and class biases is expected to provide answers to the question of why interpreting is under-appreciated.

This book, therefore, examines how the under-recognition of interpreting is tied to societal monolingualism characterised by linguistic, racial and class hierarchies from a critical sociolinguistic perspective (see Section 2.5

for details on critical sociolinguistics of interpreting). It focuses on health care interpreting as a key site of examination.

1.3 The study

This section outlines the research approaches in detail.

1.3.1 Health care interpreting as a key site of inquiry

There are three key reasons behind the book's focus on health care interpreting.

First, there is a significant dearth of research on inequality and power in health care interpreting. Most interpreting research on inequality focuses on the legal space (see Section 2.4 for details). Inequality is, however, not limited to the legal space. It is also relevant to other institutional contexts including health care. Taking some examples, patients with limited proficiency in the dominant language tend to be treated poorly, with minority patients subject to discrimination by health care providers (Hanssens et al., 2017). Furthermore, individuals who are not literate in the dominant language are excluded from potentially life-saving information, such as health and vaccine information regarding COVID-19 (Piller et al., 2020). Interpreting is generally regarded as a solution to address access inequity for vulnerable groups (Gil-Salmerón et al., 2021; see also Angermeyer, 2023). However, the normative idea of interpreting as an enabler of health equity may work to conceal problems which significantly impact vulnerable populations when trying to access health services. Considering this knowledge gap, it is important to explore biases in health care interpreting to promote access equity for minority groups.

Second, the three key foci of this book – language, race and class – are highly relevant to Australian health care, which has long been dominated by Anglo-Celtic norms and English monolingualism (see also Section 3.3). Non-white NESB populations such as Indigenous Australians have been historically discriminated within the racialised institutional structures (Durey, 2015). Furthermore, English monolingualism has dominated health care, as exemplified by the description of Australian hospitals as "unusually monolingual" (Phillips, 2016, p. 210). According to Johnstone and Kanitsaki (2008), English-related prejudice in Australian health care is so strong that biases against NESB groups including staff, nurses, patients and importantly, interpreters have been deeply internalised. The deep-seated nature of English monolingualism in Australian health care is demonstrated by the dominant attitude which treats interpreters as an economic cost, despite their obvious importance to patients unable to speak English (Johnstone & Kanitsaki, 2008). As "a social institution built on the cultural stance of the population it serves" (Henry et al., 2004, p. 518), Australian health care represents a key site to investigate institutional biases relating to other languages and speakers and their impact on interpreting.

Finally, as the first interpreting service institutionalised in Australia, health care interpreting is a key to understand the historical interplays between English monolingualism and migrant struggles (including those of interpreters) at the intersections between language, race and class. Established in 1977 following the multicultural turn of Australia, health care interpreting was a response to migrant struggles and poverty caused by language barriers, a problem compounded by the 'White Australia' policy (1901–1973). Born out of the complex social, racial and linguistic relations in Australia (see Chapter 3 for details), health care interpreting represents an ideological site to understand the exclusive roles that English has played in maintaining social hierarchies, the impact of English monolingualism on the marginalisation of other languages and speakers and its influence on shaping the public perception of interpreting.

1.3.2 Qualitative approaches

This book takes qualitative approaches, which consist of historical textual analysis and semi-structured interviews with health care interpreters. To begin with, historical textual analysis is designed to examine how English monolingualism in Australia has become tied to linguistic, racial and class hierarchies and how it has influenced and reinforced the minoritisation of interpreters and interpreting. The inquiry has been examined by following the development of the profession of health care interpreting under the evolving sociolinguistic conditions of Australia through the pre-federation period (before 1901), White Australia (1901–1973) and the development of multiculturalism since then. Data for analysis was obtained from books, journal articles, magazines and other online sources, with 'Australia', 'English monolingualism', 'interpreting', 'interpreters' and 'health care' as key words. This approach provides a baseline for understanding interpreting as an ideological site shaped by English monolingualism.

The other source of data was obtained from semi-structured interviews with health care interpreters. Participant recruitment began in early 2022 and ran through the first half of the year. Interpreters were selected if they had at least one year's experience with health care interpreting and held interpreting certification provided by the National Accreditation Authority for Translators and Interpreters (NAATI), a national governing body of translators and interpreters in Australia. The participants were recruited through two different avenues: i) an online NAATI directory which contains the contact details of all translators and interpreters in

Australia by language category and location; ii) the NSW Multicultural Health Service, which administers health care interpreting service across New South Wales. Contacts with interpreters for recruitment were made via email, and a total of 67 health care interpreters (representing 28 languages) from across Australia participated in one-on-one interviews.

All interviews were conducted via Zoom as part of social distancing measures imposed by the COVID-19 pandemic. Each interview took approximately one hour, and all were recorded on Zoom. In line with the principle of responsive interviewing (Rubin & Rubin, 2011), which aims to achieve solid, deep understanding rather than breadth, the interviews paid attention to the "complexity of multiple, overlapping and sometimes conflicting themes" (p. 35) by matching questions to participants' responses and interests. General guiding questions included perceptions and treatment of interpreting in various social and professional contexts.

The Zoom-recorded interviews were transcribed by a professional transcription service provider and the proofed interview transcripts were coded by me in NVivo. Thematic analysis proposed by Braun and Clarke (2012) served as a key analytical prism, and data analysis followed four specific steps. The first step involved data familiarisation through repeated reading of interview transcripts to identify core patterns. This was followed by the subsequent step of coding, in which data was systematically organised into distinctive meaning units. In the third step, themes were generated by considering not only the unique characteristics of individual codes but also the connections between them. The rigour of theme generation was strengthened through a constant dialogue with the data and a recursive process of comparing themes with the coded data and the entire dataset. In the final step, the generated themes were further refined, with each theme developed not only in its own right but also in relation to the other themes. Through this process, coherent and comprehensive stories emerged to provide a valuable insight into the relations between the under-appreciation of interpreting and English monolingualism.

1.3.3 Structure of the book

This book consists of seven chapters. Following this introductory chapter, Chapter 2 contextualises the key inquiries of the book by examining how monolingualism is tied to linguistic, racial and class hierarchies based on relevant literature. It also provides an overview of English monolingualism in Australia and institutional monolingualism in interpreting. The chapter concludes by discussing and highlighting the relevance of critical sociolinguistic approaches to the examination of the under-recognition of interpreting as an issue of social inequality.

Chapter 3 examines the ties between societal monolingualism and interpreting by tracing how English monolingualism has become implicated in language, racial and class biases against NESB migrants in the historical context of Australia. By following the processes by which health care interpreting began and has developed in English-monolingual Australia, the chapter explores migrant struggles caused by language barriers, societal ignorance of communication problems and the isolation of interpreting as a job for migrants by migrants. It illuminates the poor recognition of interpreting as not just a contemporary problem, but an issue strongly embedded in historical biases against other languages and speakers.

Moving on to the contemporary era, Chapter 4 investigates the impact of market monolingualism on interpreters. It examines how interpreting is treated in the interpreting market by focusing on the relations between English monolingualism and interpreting as a migrant-concentrated profession. The chapter uncovers how racial and class biases reinforce market monolingualism against migrant-background interpreters, and impact professional recognition of interpreting, especially in monetary terms. The chapter also explores how interpreters respond to market monolingualism in relation to their migrant status.

Chapter 5 examines institutional monolingualism and the ways it impacts health care interpreters working for Australian hospitals. It investigates institutional perception of interpreting at three different levels – front desk staff, doctors, and hospital systems. The chapter also explores institutional biases against patients with limited English assisted by interpreters. It specifically focuses on how institutional monolingualism represents formidable barriers to interpreters within the context of power differentials between interpreters and health care providers.

Following the examination of institutional monolingualism, Chapter 6 explores how interpreters respond to institutional monolingualism in their daily dealings with communication problems. It pays specific attention to how interpreters manage culturally unique concepts which do not easily translate into the other language within the monolingual milieu of Australian hospitals. The chapter highlights interpreting as solo work that has been naturalised and strengthened within institutional monolingualism. It also provides various suggestions from the participants to health care providers to promote awareness of interpreting, through which to achieve inter-party collaboration.

The concluding chapter revisits the research questions raised at the beginning of the book, emphasising the under-appreciation of interpreting as a manifestation of societal ignorance of other languages and speakers. It illuminates interpreting as a key site within which to examine social inequality by calling for more attention to problems with interpreting through critical sociolinguistic approaches to interpreting.

Note

1 The social recognition of interpreting relating to English as valued forms of capital in Korea is explored in Cho, *English language ideologies in Korea: Interpreting the past and present.*

References

Adoniou, M. (2018). Monolingualism in multicultural Australia: Paradoxes and challenges. In Y. K. Cha, S. H. Ham, & M. Lee (Eds.), *Routledge international handbook of multicultural education research in Asia Pacific* (pp. 272–285). Routledge.

Angelelli, C. (2004a). *Revisiting the interpreter's role: A study of conference, court and medical interpreters in Canada, Mexico and the United States*. John Benjamins Publishing.

Angelelli, C. (2004b). *Medical interpreting and cross-cultural communication*. Cambridge University Press.

Angermeyer, P. S. (2023). Translation as discrimination: Sociolinguistics and inequality in multilingual institutional contexts. *Language in Society*, *52*(5), 837–859. doi:10.1017=S0047404522000422

Aranguri, C., Davidson, B., & Ramirez, R. (2006). Patterns of communication through interpreters: A detailed sociolinguistic analysis. *Journal of General Internal Medicine*, *21*(6), 623–629.

Ayan, I. (2020). Re-thinking neutrality through emotional labour: The (in)visible work of conference interpreters. *TTR*, *33*(2), 125–146. https://doi.org/10.7202/1077714ar

Bahadir, Ş. (2017). The interpreter as observer, participant and agent of change: The irresistible entanglement between interpreting ethics, politics and pedagogy. In M. Biagini, M. S. Boyd, & C. Monacelli (Eds.), *The changing role of the interpreter* (pp. 122–145). Routledge.

Baker, M. (2009). Resisting state terror: Theorizing communities of activist translators and interpreters. In E. Beolsa (Ed.), *Globalization, political violence and translation* (pp. 222–242). Palgrave Macmillan.

Bourdieu, P. (1986). The forms of capital. In J. Richardson (Ed.), *Handbook of theory and research for the sociology of education* (pp. 96–111). Greenwood Press.

Bourdieu, P. (1990). *The logic of practice*. Polity Press.

Bourdieu, P. (1993). *Sociology in question*. Sage.

Braun, V., & Clarke, V. (2012). Thematic analysis. In H. Cooper (Ed.), *APA handbook of research methods in psychology* (pp. 57–71). APA Books.

Cho, J. (2017). *English language ideologies in Korea: Interpreting the past and present*. Springer.

Cho, J. (2021a). 'That's not how we speak': Interpreting monolingual ideologies in courtrooms. *Griffith Law Review*, *30*(1), 50–70. https://doi.org/10.1080/10383441.2021.1932234

Cho, J. (2021b). *Intercultural communication in interpreting: Power and choices*. Routledge. https://doi.org/10.4324/9781003179993

Clyne, M. (2005). *Australia's language potential.* UNSW Press.

Colley, H., & Guéry, F. (2015). Understanding new hybrid professions: Bourdieu, illusio and the case of public service interpreters. *Cambridge Journal of Education*, *45*(1), 113–131. https://doi.org/10.1080/0305764X.2014.991277

Dam, H. V. (2017). Interpreter role, ethics and norms: Linking to professionalization. In M. Biagini, M. S. Boyd, & C. Monacelli (Eds.), *The changing role of the interpreter: Contextualising norms, ethics and quality standards* (pp. 228–239). Routledge.

Darwish, A. (2005). The translation profession in Australia: Viability or survivability?. *Translation Watch Quarterly*, *1*, 82–92.

de Pedro Ricoy, R. (2010). Training public service interpreters in the UK: A fine balancing act. *The Journal of Specialised Translation*, *14*, 100–120.

D'Hayer, D. (2012). Public service interpreting and translation: Moving towards a (virtual) community of practice. *Meta*, *57*(1), 235–247. https://doi.org/10.7202/1012751ar

Diriker, E. (2003). Simultaneous conference interpreting in the Turkish printed and electronic media 1988-2003. *The Interpreters' Newsletter*, *12*, 231–243.

Du, Y., & Wang, B. (2021). A multi-dimensional analysis of the representation of conference interpreters in the Chinese media. *Translation Spaces*, *10*(2), 306–328. https://doi.org/10.1075/ts.18011.du

Durey, A. (2015). Antonio Gramsci and Pierre Bourdieu: 'Whiteness' and indigenous healthcare. In Collyer, F. (Ed.), *The Palgrave handbook of social theory in health, illness and medicine* (pp. 191–204). Palgrave Macmillan.

Gentile, P. (2016). *The interpreter's professional status. A sociological investigation into the interpreting profession* [Doctoral dissertation, Università degli Studi di Trieste]. https://arts.units.it/handle/11368/2908044

Gil-Salmerón, A., Katsas, K., Riza, E., Karnaki, P., & Linos, A. (2021). Access to healthcare for migrant patients in Europe: Healthcare discrimination and translation services. *International Journal of Environmental Research and Public Health*, *18*(15), 1–14. https://doi.org/10.3390/ijerph18157901

Giustini, D. (2016). Conference interpreting as a social practice. A Bourdieusian theoretical approach. *Interpreting and Translation Studies: The Journal of the Japan Association for Interpreting and Translation Studies*, *16*, 107–124. https://doi.org/10.50837/its.1606

Giustini, D. (2022). Haken conference interpreters in Japan: Exploring status through the sociology of work and of professions. *Interpreting and Society*, *2*(1), 3–31. https://doi.org/10.1177/27523810211057447

Hale, S. (2007). *Community interpreting.* Springer.

Halley, M. (2019). Interpreting as ideologically-structured action: Collective identity between activist interpreters and protesters. *New Voices in Translation Studies*, *20*(1), 54–85. https://doi.org/10.14456/nvts.2019.4

Hanssens, L. G., Detollenaere, J. D., Van Pottelberge, A., Baert, S., & Willems, S. J. (2017). Perceived discrimination in primary healthcare in Europe: Evidence from the cross-sectional QUALICOPC study. *Health & Social Care in the Community*, *25*(2), 641–651. https://doi.org/10.1111/hsc.12353

Henry, B. R., Houston, S., & Mooney, G. H. (2004). Institutional racism in Australian healthcare: A plea for decency. *Medical Journal of Australia*, *180*(10), 517–520.

Hlavac, J. (2015). Formalizing community interpreting standards: A cross-national comparison of testing systems, certification conventions and recent ISO guidelines. *International Journal of Interpreter Education*, *7*(2), 21–38.

Inghilleri, M. (2003). Habitus, field and discourse: Interpreting as a socially situated activity. *Target. International Journal of Translation Studies*, *15*(2), 243–268. https://doi.org/10.1075/target.15.2.03ing

Inghilleri, M. (Ed.) (2005). Bourdieu and the sociology of translation and interpreting [Special issue]. *The Translator, 11*(2).

Johnstone, M. J., & Kanitsaki, O. (2008). Cultural racism, language prejudice and discrimination in hospital contexts: An Australian study. *Diversity and Equality in Health and Care*, *5*(1), 19–30.

Lee, J., Choi, M., Huh, J., & Chang, A. (2016). Community interpreting services by marriage migrants for marriage migrants in South Korea. *Perspectives*, *24*(2), 179–200. https://doi.org/10.1080/0907676X.2015.1052524

Mason, I., & Ren, W. (2012). Power in face-to-face interpreting events. *Translation and Interpreting Studies*, *7*(2), 234–253. http://doi10.1075/tis.7.2.08mas

Mikkelson, H. (1996). The professionalization of community interpreting. In M. O'Keeffe (Ed.), *Global vision: Proceedings of the 37th Annual Conference of the American Translators Association* (pp. 77–89). American Translators Association.

Phillips, C. B. (2016). Improving health outcomes for linguistically diverse patients. *The Medical Journal of Australia*, *204*, 209–210.

Piller, I., Torsh, H., & Smith-Khan, L. (2023). Securing the borders of English and Whiteness. *Ethnicities*, *23*(5), 706–725. https://doi.org/10.1177/14687968211052610

Piller, I., Zhang, J., & Li, J. (2020). Linguistic diversity in a time of crisis: Language challenges of the COVID-19 pandemic. *Multilingua*, *39*(5), 503–515. https://doi.org/10.1515/multi-2020-0136

Roy, C., & Metzger, M. (2014). Researching signed language interpreting research through a sociolinguistic lens. *Translation & Interpreting: The International Journal of Translation and Interpreting Research*, *6*(1), 158–176. https://doi.org/ti.106201.2014.a09

Rubin, H. J., & Rubin, I. S. (2011). *Qualitative interviewing: The art of hearing data*. Sage.

Simeoni, D. (1998). The pivotal status of the translator's habitus. *Target. International Journal of Translation Studies*, *10*(1), 1–39. https://doi.org/10.1075/target.10.1.02sim

Tekgül, D. (2020). Faith-related interpreting as emotional labour: A case study at a Protestant Armenian church in Istanbul. *Perspectives*, *28*(1), 43–57. https://doi.org/10.1080/0907676X.2019.1641527

Ulaş, A. P., & Gündüz, A. (2020). A bourdieusian perspective on the public service interpreters working at the non-governmental organizations. *Çeviribilim ve Uygulamaları Dergisi*, *28*, 144–176. https://doi.org/10.37599/ceviri.675408

Valero Garcés, C., & Gauthier Blasi, L. (2010). Bourdieu and public service interpreting and translation: Towards a social theory in PSIT. *MonTI. Monografías de Traducción e Interpretación*, 2, 97–117. http://doi:10.6035/MonTI.2010.2.5

Wadensjö, C. (2014). *Interpreting as interaction*. Routledge. https://doi.org/10.4324/9781315842318

2 Monolingual understanding of multilingualism

2.1 Rethinking monolingualism

To examine how the under-appreciation of interpreting relates to the linguistic, racial and class hierarchies in English-monolingual Australia, it is important to establish the ties that link monolingualism with those hierarchies. Monolingualism is a frequent topic of investigation in sociolinguistics, yet the concept remains rather elusive. At a micro-individual level, defining monolingualism involves the fundamental questions of language, language proficiency and speakers (Ellis, 2006, 2008). In the most basic sense, a monolingual person is one who speaks only one language. This, however, quickly leads to complex questions such as how monolingual one should be to qualify, what variety of language, i.e., standard versus dialect, one should speak to be a monolingual and how proficient one should be in the language to be eligible as a monolingual speaker. Usual responses to these questions would be that a monolingual is someone who speaks only one language, which is a standard variety, as their mother tongue (from birth) without any proficiency in other languages at all. This is because of the strong association between monolingualism and native speakers, according to which a monolingual is a native speaker, and a native speaker is also a monolingual (Cook, 1999; Ellis, 2016).

At a macro-ideological level, monolingualism commonly refers to a narrow view of language which sees one language variety as superior to other varieties (Piller, 2016a). As an "ideology which implies that clarity, logic and unity depend on the adoption of a monoglot standard variety in public discourse" (Blackledge, 2000, p. 27), monolingualism is strongly grounded in the legitimacy and superiority of one specific language variety. The exclusionary nature of monolingualism is succinctly explained by Ellis (2006, 2008) who has identified three important ideological dimensions of monolingualism.

The first representation of monolingualism concerns the *naturalisation of monolingualism as a norm* or the "unmarked case" (Ellis, 2008, p. 314).

DOI: 10.4324/9781032614854-2

As a traditionally dominant ideology tied to national identity, monolingualism is normalised as a symbol of a nation throughout the process by which the public accepts and internalises the superiority of one language over the others (see also Bourdieu, 1990). This aspect of monolingualism is said to be common in powerful societies (e.g., countries in Europe) which have fully embraced the ideology of 'one nation, one language' in the process of building modern nations. In this representation, other languages are deemed to be incompatible with the nation-state characterised by linguistic homogeneity and, therefore, lack legitimacy.

Second, monolingualism entails *limited opportunities and potential of both individuals and societies*. Knowledge of other languages can bring a range of benefits such as greater cognitive flexibility, creative problem-solving skills, enhanced employability and other personal benefits, which, in turn, translate into social benefits. Despite such benefits, multilingualism remains an exception in many societies including Australia. Knowing only one language is said to not only reduce material benefits such as employment opportunities but also limit our vision and constrain our understanding (see also Piller, 2016b). Reduced opportunities from being a monolingual have direct implications on social development, hence the argument that monolingualism limits human potential and societies.

The third and final representation of monolingualism is *monolingualism as an insidious state bordering on a pathological disorder*. In this representation, monolingualism is argued to be a product of deliberate political orchestration to exclude various groups of populations as well as an outcome of misguided education policies which fail to prioritise language learning. A resultant lack of language awareness works to stereotype and stigmatise bilinguals as deficient speakers of the dominant language, while valorising monolinguals as native speakers of the privileged language. As people who are monolingual tend to be in powerful positions, their limited understanding of how languages work and how they differ may lead to a denial of important resources and opportunities for significant portions of populations. Persistent refusal to accept bilingualism as a normal part of our increasingly multilingual world is pathological, a state which privileged monolingual groups are intent to defend by framing bilingualism negatively.

As such, monolingualism can be seen as both a state and a mode of operation characterised by the binary logic of inclusion versus exclusion, shaped by and naturalised through historical, social and political relations with language which dominate our contemporary consciousness and practice of language.

The hegemonic nature of monolingual ideologies is well exemplified by English monolingualism in English-speaking Anglophone countries. In the case of the U.S., monolingual English ideologies tied to nationalism and social integration have continued to dominate the public psyche. There, linguistic diversity is framed as a divisive force through its history of mass migration (Wiley & Lukes, 1996). Migrants' retention of the original language was seen as disloyalty to the nation, with true patriotism constructed as being a monolingual in English (Leeman, 2018).

In the case of the U.K., accent biases relating to standard English are particularly strong due to its long history of accent-based class hierarchies. People who can speak 'Queen's English' enjoy accent prestige, whereas those speaking English with ethnic minority accents are subject to stereotypes that see them as less educated and socioeconomically inferior (Levon et al., 2022). In a study regarding discrimination against migrants in British workplaces (Goulden, 2022), for example, it was noted that speakers having African accents are seen to be an archetype of refugees and poor migrants who are assumed to be uneducated, unskilled, unintelligent and untrustworthy within the workplace. The monoglot ways of treating other languages and their speakers highlight 'monolingualism as ethnocentrism', according to which language-based discrimination is naturalised and institutionalised (Lippi-Green, 1994).

While the discriminatory nature of monolingualism is evident in the extant scholarship, it is important to note that a focus has been placed on the linguistic aspects of monolingualism, with less attention paid to racial and class orders. The workings of monolingualism against other languages as well as their speakers raise the question of how racial and class biases interact with linguistic biases to inform the ways in which monolingualism operates. The next section examines this very question by focusing on how language, race and class are inseparable from one another to serve as a metaphorical border in a collective sense.

2.2 Borders in language, race and class

In her seminal paper *Language and borders*, anthropologist Bonnie Urciuoli (1995) illuminates how language differences signify ethnic or national origins of speakers, which together act as borders in a metaphorical sense. In such categorisations, language is seen as an exclusive possession which belongs to certain individuals and groups, and borders can be politicised to reinforce existing power relations. Language-based borders are not just metaphorical. They can also be physical, and can be clearly exemplified by national borders informed by the concept of modern nation-state and monolingual ideology.

As discussed above, monolingualism values one language variety over others and tends to perceive other languages as threats to national, social and political integration. The superior versus inferior binary in monolingualism dates to 19th-century Europe characterised by the political movement towards a nation-state. The concept of a nation-state hardly existed in Medieval Europe, with national sentiment carrying little meaning in most European countries (May, 2017). As the monolingual nation-state emerged as a political ideal, the group that became dominant pushed their language as the national language, consolidating language as a demarcating borderline (Billig, 1995).

Language as borders and a marker of a nation-state culminated at the Versailles Peace Conference following the First World War, in which the principle of the nation-state and language was upheld as a basis for determining nationality and/or ethnicity (Smolicz, 1984). Through the process of nation-state building, the ideology of 'one nation, one language' was firmly entrenched, with language serving not only practical but also symbolic purposes of defining the essence of the nation. Languages that did not fit the imagined nationhood were simplified and erased through linguistic hierarchising. Those who had power to impose their language as a norm did so by appealing to the alleged superiority of the language, which, in turn, relegated other varieties to 'dialects' or 'jargons' of the uneducated mass (Wiley, 1996). The development of printing and the mass circulation of printed words further contributed to the privileging of the dominant language over other varieties (Ellis et al., 2010).

The dominant variety acquired the privileged status of a 'standard language', a sterile form of language without any trace of 'corruptible' elements (e.g., accent). This view of linguistic purity is most evident in standard language ideology, which is defined as "a bias toward an abstracted, idealized and homogeneous spoken language which is imposed and maintained by dominant bloc institutions" (Lippi-Green, 1994, p. 67). As a product of monolingual ideology, standard language ideology is used to justify positioning speakers of other languages at the lower rung of a social hierarchy, while elevating people capable of producing the dominant variety as superior speakers of the language.

As such, language serves as class borders. The relations between language and class are powerfully explained by Bourdieu (1977a, 1977b, 1979, 1990, 1991), who paid specific attention to the role of language in producing and reproducing class relations. The theory of linguistic market (1993) demonstrates that as products, all speeches and, by extension, all speakers are valuated in an abstract sense of a linguistic market. Bourdieu notes that in any society, there is a language which is more dominant than others and, with hardly any exceptions, the dominant language is the language of the dominant group. For the dominant language to be recognised as the only language of authority, the linguistic market must be unified, so that the dichotomy between the dominant and dominated languages is upheld and remains unchallenged.

To maintain the unity of the market, the relation of linguistic production endows speakers capable of producing a legitimate product with more value and acknowledgement, compared with people unable to perform the same feat. Bourdieu argues that the processes by which a certain language variety is established as a dominant language are determined not only sociohistorically but also along social class lines. That is, the dominant language works as an exclusive marker of class legitimacy, reinforcing the 'distinction' (Bourdieu, 1984) of its speakers, while excluding others. Once a certain language is established as the language of power, pursuit of the language as a key to social mobility follows. The standard language ideology in the U.S., for example, promotes monolingualism by normalising the acquisition of standard English as a key to mobility (Collins, 1991). In this way, language strengthens and reinforces class-based borders.

Class is inseparable from race (Bannerji, 2005), and language- and class-based borders can extend to racial borders too. The ties between language and race are most powerfully demonstrated by raciolinguistic theory (Flores & Rosa, 2015; Rosa & Flores, 2017). The raciolinguistic perspective posits the "co-naturalization of language and race as a process of *raciolinguistic enregisterment* whereby linguistic and racial forms are jointly constructed as sets" (Rosa & Flores, 2017, p. 11, emphasis in original). Grounded in the project of modernity led by European colonialism, raciolinguistic ideologies were used to justify the binary between Europeanness and non-Europeanness, whiteness and non-whiteness, and European languages and other languages. As two central keys to European colonial domination, language and race were hierarchised according to the standards set by the rulers, resulting in linguistic and racial subjugations of non-white and non-European populations.

It might be tempting to dismiss the racial and linguistic logics as irrelevant to the contemporary era, yet the raciolinguistic binary still impacts the modern perception of language and speakers. All too often, people 'see' accent in speech (see Rosa, 2019). Taking some examples, Kutlu (2023) demonstrates that people's evaluation of linguistic output is influenced by the colour of the speaker. When American English and Indian English speakers were presented with South Asian faces versus white faces, listeners judged speech presented with coloured faces as more accented compared with that presented with white faces, regardless of the type of English. 'Raciolinguistic borders' (Cushing, 2023) impact racial minority populations in education in which aspirant teachers from minority backgrounds are expected to modify their speech to be accepted as legitimate professionals.

As such, language, class and race are strongly interconnected, indicating that monolingualism is not just about language but is strongly tied to racial and class relations. Existing structures and prejudice against minority groups are normalised through various strategies, with some less explicit than others. Examples of explicit strategies include education policies that fail to prioritise language learning and school tests that disadvantage students from minority backgrounds (Ellis, 2006). Those that are less explicit tend to be more insidious due to the very lack of visibility. These strategies involve political ideological orchestration which establishes monolingualism as the only norm by manipulating public ideas about language. Systems and processes that have the veneer of democracy make it harder to problematise dominant practices, in which 'consensus' on monolingual ideologies and practices is achieved and the worldview of the elite class becomes universalised (Woolard, 1998).

This state in which the ideas of the ruling group are accepted as a universal truth is referred to as *doxa* in Bourdieu's theory (Bourdieu, 1990). Keeping dominant ideologies in a *doxic* state that is unquestioned and unquestionable requires continuous and active participation of subaltern groups in ideological reproduction processes and *symbolic power* represents a key to understanding the 'voluntary' participation of the subjugated. Defined as "invisible power which can be exercised only with the complicity of those who do not want to know that they are subject to it or even that they themselves exercise it" (Bourdieu, 1991, p. 164), symbolic power helps the naturalisation and spread of dominant ideologies, creating fictitious images of social integration and harmony. Precisely how the projected social world is best suited to the interests of the dominant group is, however, concealed, as it is recognised or *misrecognised* by the dominated who are unable to realise the very exclusionary nature of the normative truth. This process of manipulation by which the boundaries of *doxa* are enforced is referred to as *symbolic violence*, which is "exercised upon a social agent with his or her own complicity" (Bourdieu & Wacquant, 1992, p. 167).

As a country long dominated by English, Australia represents a key site to examine how the practice of linguistic border-making interplays with class and racial hierarchies to create a *doxic* state of English monolingualism.

2.3 English monolingualism in Australia

English monolingualism in Australia has been most popularly described as a "monolingual mindset" (Clyne, 2005), which refers to a tendency that sees "everything in terms of a single language [English]" (p. 348). While around 300 different languages are spoken in Australia, those languages are literally invisible due to the domination of English. Clyne (2008) argues that a monolingual mindset is manifested in three main areas. First, it sees monolingualism as the norm and knowing more than one language as an exception. It further regards plurilingualism as deviant, unnecessary, undesirable or even dangerous. Second, a monolingual mindset fails to understand the ties between skills in one language and those in others. Third, beliefs in monolingualism are reflected in social and educational planning, which, in turn, strengthens existing monolingual attitudes.

In his seminal book entitled *Community languages: The Australian experience* (1991), Clyne examines the historical processes by which Australia has become a "multilingual society with a monolingual mindset" (Clyne, 2008, p. 349). It indicates that English monolingualism is deeply implicated in key historical issues including national identity, migration, economic development and politics and has strong resonance in contemporary Australia (see Chapter 3 for details).

The endurance of a monolingual mindset can be understood through the concept of "monolingual habitus" (Gogolin, 1997), which is based on Bourdieu's theory of habitus. As a system of durable disposition (Bourdieu, 1977b), habitus is acquired from socially structured space and is shaped by past social conditions that inform current practice. Social life is not just a summation of mechanic reactions by individuals to structures, yet agents regenerate the structures of which they are the product (Bourdieu, 1997b). As a structuring mechanism, habitus is both conscious and unconscious, the latter of which is evident in the notion of *doxa* (see also Section 2.2). Conditioned in the 'objective' structures, agents including both the dominated and the dominant (mis)recognise relations of dominance as common sense, which, in turn, strengthens dominant practices. Misrecognised this way, habitus reinforces the undisputed acceptance of the daily lifeworld (Bourdieu & Wacquant, 1992).

If applied to language, habitus explains the uncontested acceptance of the linguistic relations of dominance. Defined as the "deep-seated habit of assuming monolingualism as the norm in a nation" (Gogolin, 1997, p. 41), monolingual habitus significantly influences individual and group behaviours relating to language. Gogolin illustrates this point with the 'professional habitus' of teachers at German schools in which establishing monolingualism in the official language through teaching is an "imperative in a teacher's professional ethos" (p. 42). Teaching methods which " 'appeal to a feeling for language' " (p. 48, emphasis in original) for immigrant students who have neither implicit linguistic knowledge nor appropriate learning techniques are clearly exclusionary. They are not, however, recognised as such within the professional community embedded in monolingual ideologies.

If applied to Australia, a monolingual habitus or a monolingual mindset has historically excluded and disadvantaged non-English-speaking background (hereafter 'NESB') populations. According to Al Grassby (1984), who was known as the "father of Australian multiculturalism" (Whitlam government minister Al Grassby dies, 2005), the term 'migrant', be it migrant children, migrant languages or migrant cultures, has essentially meant non-white and NESB in Australia, a label that has been stigmatised through recurring racism against migrants throughout Australian history. Grassby argues that Australians whose discriminatory behaviours had been permitted and even encouraged throughout individual upbringing, schooling and social interactions continued to see prejudice against migrants as normal even after the country became officially multicultural.

Discrimination against NESB populations in Australia was not just racial and class-based but also linguistic. Grassby (1984) noted that during the period of White Australia, not being able to speak English well was considered a 'handicap'. Hundreds of thousands of Australian-born children speaking a language other than English as their first language were made monolinguals through school education delivered through biased teachers and textbooks. As part of the social homogeneity project, English monolingualism was a marker of Australianness tied to whiteness, rendering other languages and speakers a threat to social unity (see Chapter 3 for details). This suggests that a monolingual mindset is not just about language but relates to racial and class hierarchies in the historical context of Australia.

The myth of homogeneity has had an enduring impact on contemporary Australia too, as exemplified by the continued dominance of English and whiteness. Although Australia does not have an official language, English serves as a de-facto national language (Cho, 2024). The legacy of Anglo-Celtic cultures still dominates the society (Forrest et al., 2021) and 'white privilege' is a persistent problem (Elias et al., 2021). Under such circumstances, NESB populations in contemporary Australia continue to experience disadvantages including denial of employment and promotion (Colic-Peisker, 2011; Hawthorne, 1997), marginalisation at school (Riggs & Due, 2011) and social isolation (Cho, 2021b; Ip et al., 2007).

While proficiency in English is regarded as a ticket to social participation in Australia, the binary logic of inclusion versus exclusion in English monolingualism goes deeper than mere proficiency in English: it is not just any English but so-called 'standard Australian English' that serves as the norm for inclusion. Standard Australian English refers to an idealised form of English "in terms of its *logic, history, or aesthetics*" (Tankosić et al., 2021, p. 1783, emphasis in original). NESB populations who *can* speak English tend to be judged on how close or further they sound from the standard norm (Tankosić & Dovchin, 2023). The further they sound, the more they suffer in various forms. Forms of suffering range from language-based inferiority complexes, anxiety, reduced confidence and self-esteem to emotional reactions (e.g., outbursts of crying) (Dovchin, 2020; Dryden & Dovchin, 2024). Importantly, NESB migrants unable to produce the socially sanctioned speech are demonstrably non-white and tend to occupy low social status. This only indicates the racialised and class-based dimensions of language in English-monolingual Australia.

The internalised state of linguistic, class and racial hierarchies in English monolingualism in Australia raises a question. Does the normalised state of those hierarchies influence a space which is supposed to be neutral and unbiased yet involves other languages and speakers at all times – interpreting – and, if so, how? The next section examines the relations between interpreting and monolingualism by focusing on interpreter-mediated institutional settings.

2.4 Institutional monolingualism in interpreting

Australia is the first country to officially introduce community interpreting. Its launch of the health care interpreting services in 1977 was the world's first. Following their introduction, Australia established a centralised certification system which governs translators and interpreters, also for the first time in the world. Furthermore, the country has provided free interpreting (and translation) services for linguistic minorities since 1973 and is regarded as a global leader of translation and interpreting (Bischoff, 2020).

The provision of free language services is, indeed, what distinguishes Australia from the other Anglo English-speaking countries which do not have comparable systems. Rather than seeing translation and interpreting as an enabler of social integration, politicians in certain parts of the world see language services as disincentives for migrants to learn the dominant language (Pokorn & Čibej, 2017). This negative view of translation and interpreting stems from the ignorance of challenges relating to language learning, the success of which is seen to be solely dependent on migrants' individual efforts when it is, in fact, determined by a variety of factors including age, education, gender, religion and social networks (Adserà & Pytliková, 2016; Rida & Milton, 2001).

While Australia is clearly setting an example in terms of language services, the existence of the system may not automatically translate into the intended goal of enhanced equity for vulnerable populations. The extant research which focuses on legal interpreting reveals that monolingual biases impact everyday interpreting practice in Australia. In a broad sense, three specific dimensions of institutional monolingualism bear strong resemblance to societal monolingualism characterised by biases against other languages and speakers.

First, similar to societal monolingualism, institutional monolingualism in interpreting recognises the dominant language as the only legitimate language. Taking interpreter-assisted Australian court proceedings as an example, Eades (2003) found out that only the English utterances are recorded in the official transcripts and the other language is not included for record keeping. The court's failure to record non-English testimony can bring about serious consequences to trial outcomes if the court-appointed interpreter misinterprets and no one notices. Misinterpreting is more likely to occur when the interpreter provides simultaneous interpreting of court proceedings for the NESB defendant. This method is more cognitively demanding and error-prone than consecutive interpreting (see Angermeyer, 2015). The prioritisation of English is also evident in refugee interviews in Australia in which decision-makers are permitted to assess the quality of interpreting output regardless of their bilingual skills (see Smith-Khan, 2017). As bilingual skills are not required to assess interpreting output, many decision-makers are likely to evaluate interpreting quality based on the English output only. This reflects inadequate institutional understanding of interpreting and language practice governed by English.

Second, institutional monolingualism in interpreting upholds the 'one nation, one language' ideology which has dominated modern nation-states. Taking Arabic as an example, Arabic serves as the official language of many countries in the Arab region. Spoken forms of Arabic across the countries in the region, however, significantly differ, with only the written form of Arabic comprehensible to all Arab countries. Among localised spoken varieties, some vernaculars (e.g., Sudanese-Arabic) differ to the point that they are not mutually comprehensible. Such linguistic diversity is, however, not properly understood in the Australian judicial space. Cho's (2021b) research illustrates how an 'Arabic' interpreter speaking a different variety of Arabic is often assigned to Arabic-speaking court participants in Australia. Linguistic discordance between the court-appointed interpreter and the lay court participant can cause misinterpreting and can lead to unfair judicial outcomes for linguistic minorities (see Cho, 2021a, 2021b). As such, institutional monolingualism is identified as a potential cause of inequality for vulnerable populations.

Third, institutional monolingualism in interpreting categorises speakers between those who can speak 'our' language and those who cannot, bearing resemblance to the 'us-them' binary embedded in societal monolingualism. According to this logic, linguistic minorities are seen as monolinguals in their language unable to speak the dominant language at all and are expected to behave in a way that fits the stereotype of monolingual minority speakers (Cho, 2021b; see also Angermeyer, 2015). Contrary to such beliefs, however, many lay court participants can speak the dominant language, yet they resort to interpreters to ensure accurate representation due to complex legal terminology and discourses (Angermeyer, 2015; Cho, 2021b). When linguistic minorities inadvertently display their bilingual abilities in interpreter-mediated court proceedings, courts tend to see their conduct as deception and suspect that bilingual participants pretend not to understand the dominant language to be deceptive.

The 'us-them' distinction applies to interpreters too. In Australian courtrooms, it is reported that legal professionals tend to treat testimony coming from interpreters speaking 'standard Australian English' as more credible, compared to interpreters speaking with a foreign accent (Cho, 2021a). This is problematic because many interpreters in migrant-receiving countries have migrant backgrounds and speak the dominant language with an accent (Hale et al., 2011). As linguistic minority participants can represent themselves only through the words of interpreters, the 'accented' speech of interpreters may impact the ways in which credibility is perceived and assessed by legal professionals. This situation also illustrates the racialised and class-based dimensions of monolingualism in the space of interpreting in which most interpreters are migrants.

The examination of institutional monolingualism in Australian legal interpreting highlights the ways that interpreting, which is generally believed to be an enabler of access equity, is vulnerable to biases against other languages and speakers. It also illuminates the institutional space of interpreting as "permeable to the mandates of the society" (Angelelli, 2004, p. 9), highlighting that institutional monolingualism does not exist in a vacuum yet operates in layered spatiality in which macro-level ideologies impact institutional practice.

While the extant body of research provides valuable insights into institutional monolingualism in interpreting, the overview identifies several research gaps.

First, research on monolingualism in interpreting has exclusively focused on legal contexts; hardly any research examines monolingualism in other interpreting contexts (see also Section 1.3.1). The strong impact of societal monolingualism on institutional monolingualism, as illustrated above, suggests that societal monolingualism may not just influence legal spaces yet may also operate in other interpreting settings. This book extends the existing research on monolingualism in interpreting contexts into health care interpreting, which is critical to ensure the health and wellbeing of marginalised populations.

Second, the vulnerability of the interpreting space to societal monolingualism raises an important question as to the nature of monolingualism in interpreting. The extant research approaches institutional monolingualism in interpreting as a predominantly linguistic problem, yet, as discussed in the previous sections of this chapter, monolingual biases are not just about language but also relate to class and racial biases. If interpreting is susceptible to institutional monolingualism which is itself tied to societal monolingualism, it can be posited that not only linguistic hierarchies but also racial and class hierarchies are at work in the interpreting space. It is, therefore, necessary to examine monolingualism in interpreting from a holistic perspective which accounts for language, race and class.

Third, there is a significant lack of research on how interpreters respond to monolingualism. The emerging body of sociologically-informed research highlights dilemmas experienced by interpreters torn between dispositions and positions (see Inghilleri, 2003, 2005), yet these are not specific to monolingualism tied to linguistic, racial and class hierarchies. Furthermore, the extant work focuses on legal interpreters, leaving room to examine interpreters' agency in other interpreting settings. In this regard, this book focuses on interpreters' responses to monolingualism from the perspectives of health care interpreters.

The next section situates these lines of inquiries within the theoretical framework of critical sociolinguistics.

2.5 Interpreting from a critical sociolinguistic perspective

To investigate the relations between the under-appreciation of interpreting and monolingualism, this book adopts a critical sociolinguistic perspective. Critical sociolinguistics is classified as a branch of sociolinguistics, itself an umbrella term "covering all kinds of investigations into how language matters, socially, politically and economically" (Heller et al., 2018, p. 2). What distinguishes critical sociolinguistics from sociolinguistics is its concern for linguistic inequality and power (Mesthrie, 2000). By asking "what resources are important to whom, and how the social processes that we examine have consequences" (Heller et al., 2018, p. 2), critical sociolinguistics concerns "processes by which systems of social inequality are created and sustained" (Tollefson, 2006, p. 43) specifically in relation to languages and their speakers. In this regard, critical sociolinguistic approaches are distinguished from descriptive approaches to language research for they challenge "the idea of objectivist sociolinguistic research" (Pietikäinen, 2016, p. 264).

Interpreting is generally regarded as a solution to inequality experienced by linguistic minorities, yet this view has been increasingly challenged in critical sociolinguistics (see Angermeyer, 2015, 2023; Berk-Seligson, 2017; Blommaert, 2009; Eades, 2003 for example). The extant work highlights power differentials in interpreting settings, inadequate institutional understandings about interpreting and institutional monolingualism as significant problems which impact interpreters' work. The relative powerlessness of interpreters strongly figures in the studies, yet little attention has been paid to why interpreters are treated as powerless despite the essential roles that they play in promoting access equity and social inclusion of linguistic minorities. The powerlessness of interpreters has been examined in relation to powerful counterparts with which interpreters work, primarily legal professionals (see Colley & Guéry, 2015; Mason & Ren, 2012), yet this question has hardly been situated within the context of societal monolingualism in which interpreters represent minority groups subject to linguistic, racial and class hierarchies.

For the purpose of this book, 'class' is defined as social stratification systems which "promote inequality in society" (Milroy, 1999, p. 236). 'Race' follows Milroy's (1999) approach that sees 'race' and 'ethnicity' as interchangeable in socially-oriented research because both involve minority groups and their struggles. In other words, race is "closely associated with ethnicity, in that it refers to physical characteristics which are treated as ethnically significant" (1999, p. 237). As for 'language', the book follows Heller's definition which sees language as "a set of resources which circulate in unequal ways in social networks and discursive spaces, and whose meaning and value are socially constructed within the constraints of social organizational processes, under specific historical conditions" (Heller, 2007, p. 2). This definition highlights three important dimensions of language which intersect with class and race and inform the approach and structure of the book.

First, the understanding of "language as a set of resources which circulate in unequal ways in social networks and discursive spaces" emphasises *social inequality relating to language*. Language as a site of inequality affecting vulnerable populations is, indeed, the central concern of critical sociolinguistics (see Baugh, 2018; Blackledge, 2006; Heller et al., 2018; Piller, 2016b; Singh, 1996; Van Parijs, 2011 for some examples). Social inequality relating to language, however, remains significantly underexplored in community interpreting, despite its obvious relevance to the issue. While institutional monolingualism in interpreting is said to be tied to societal monolingualism (see Inghilleri, 2003), 'the social' often remains vague, leaving room to explore the specific sociolinguistic conditions in which interpreting is situated.

This approach builds on the emerging body of work which focuses on the minority aspects of interpreters. Paying attention to the racial profiles of black sign language interpreters, Obasi (2013) shows that black sign language interpreters in the U.K. tend to be negatively stereotyped by clients and agencies as less professional and junior compared with white interpreters. Black interpreters are also found to be marginalised within the professional community of sign language interpreting which has been overwhelmingly white (see also Ford, 2021). Disadvantages against interpreters from minority backgrounds are demonstrated in Angerrmeyer's (2023) research which reveals that the professionalisation of interpreting services is only available for popular languages or certain standard varieties. As other language varieties are predominantly languages of small ethnic groups which tend to be low in social status, interpreters speaking those languages are disadvantaged due to the very absence of opportunities for professional recognition. These examples highlight that interpreters are not immune to social biases against minority groups, and this book explores how the specific linguistic, racial and class biases in English-monolingual Australia impact interpreters in various social and professional spaces including health care institutions and the interpreting market.

Second, language "whose meaning and value are socially constructed within the constraints of social organizational processes" indicates the *socially constructed nature of language attitudes within societal power relations*. The concept of language ideology is most relevant to understand socially held meanings attached to language. Originally developed by Silverstein (1979), language ideology is defined as "any sets of beliefs about language articulated by the users as a rationalization or justification of perceived language structure and use" (p. 193). While this pioneering work focuses on beliefs about language at an individual level, which yet relates to social structures, the concept has been increasingly applied to social inequality. A key example is Piller's (2015) conceptualisation of language ideology as "a bridge between linguistic and social structure as they rationalize and justify social inequality as an outcome of linguistic difference" (p. 1). This highlights how language ideology is leveraged by the dominant group to sustain and also to mask social inequality.

If applied to interpreting, language ideology raises the important questions of what specific meanings are attached to the dominant language vis-à-vis other languages, and how social views of language influence interpreting as both profession and practice. While language is undoubtedly the central element of interpreting, the specific relations between the perception of interpreting and a socially constructed ideology of language remain significantly under-explored. As linguistic power relations often involve class and race, it is important to examine how socially ascribed meanings attached to English intersect with race and class in interpreting in Australia.

Relatedly and finally, the meanings and value attached to language "under specific historical conditions" highlight *language as a sociohistorical construct*. It emphasises the importance of looking locally to understand how English monolingualism arose and evolved under the constantly changing sociohistorical and sociolinguistic conditions of Australia characterised by linguistic, racial and class hierarchies. The dominance of English in Australia has been well documented, particularly by Clyne (1991, 2005), yet the question of race and class in English monolingualism remains significantly under-explored. This effort will benefit from an emerging raciolinguistic perspective on interpreting, which highlights the historical boundedness of language and race in interpreting (see Flores, 2023).

Flores argues that translation and interpreting founded on the colonial logics have reproduced the colonial biases, yet there is hardly any relevant work in Australian context. This book, therefore, focuses on interpreting as a key site to examines the processes by which English monolingualism has intersected with racial and class biases within the historical context of Australia.

Through the approaches outlined above, this book aims to help us to understand how unequal relations arise under what conditions to become what they are, with interpreting as a key prism to understand the specific social field in question.

2.6 Summary

This chapter has outlined how language, class and race are not separable, indicating monolingualism is not just a linguistic but also a racial and class-based construct. It suggests that this aspect of monolingualism is particularly relevant to Australia, considering the role of English monolingualism in managing and controlling linguistic diversity and NESB migrants throughout its history. The chapter also examines institutional monolingualism in interpreter-mediated legal communication, emphasising the vulnerability of interpreting to macro-monolingual ideologies. It concludes by proposing a critical sociolinguistic perspective on interpreting by reframing interpreting as a sociolinguistic space in which interpreters are situated as minority groups subject to linguistic, racial and class biases. Based on the discussions of this chapter, the following four inquiries are identified.

First, *what are the specific sociohistorical conditions which have shaped the development of interpreting in Australia*? As noted, the ties between sociolinguistic conditions and interpreting remain significantly under-explored, and this book pays attention to the sociohistorical and sociolinguistic conditions of Australia to understand how the local particularities have influenced the development of health care interpreting. Forming Chapter 3, the answer lies in its specific examination of how English monolingualism has intersected with the evolution of interpreting within the Australian migration context characterised by linguistic, racial and class hierarchies.

Second, *how do such hierarchies impact interpreters as minorities?* The extant research on interpreting tends to focus on interpreters as professionals involved in interpreting processes. Limited effort has been taken to understand interpreters as agents having their own social profiles (see Section 1.2.1). Chapter 4, therefore, approaches interpreters as bilingual migrant workers by focusing on working conditions in the Australian interpreting market. It examines the specific racial and class dimensions of interpreting in the market operating under English monolingualism.

Third, *how do the workings of institutional monolingualism impact interpreters in health care*? Shifting attention from legal interpreting to health care interpreting, Chapter 5 examines institutional perceptions of interpreters in the case of Australian health care and how those perceptions impact the actual treatment and work of interpreters. Focusing on the racial and class dimensions of English monolingualism within Australian health care, the chapter seeks to identify specific institutional practices which impact interpreting and interpreters.

Finally, *how do interpreters respond to institutional monolingualism?* This question is answered in Chapter 6 by focusing on the aspect of interpreters as minorities working for minorities. It explores how this minority aspect influences the ways in which interpreters engage with the profession itself and also with daily professional practice within the monolingual milieu of Australian hospitals. The chapter also highlights areas for improvement to enhance collaboration between interpreters and healthcare practitioners.

References

Adserà, A., & Pytliková, M. (2016). Language and migration. In V. Ginsburgh & S. Weber (Eds.), *The Palgrave handbook of economics and language* (pp. 342–372). Palgrave Macmillan.

Angelelli, C. (2004). *Medical interpreting and cross-cultural communication.* Cambridge University Press.

Angermeyer, P. S. (2015). *Speak English or what?: Codeswitching and interpreter use in New York City courts.* Oxford University Press.

Angermeyer, P. S. (2023). Translation as discrimination: Sociolinguistics and inequality in multilingual institutional contexts. *Language in Society*, *52*(5), 837–859. http://doi:10.1017/S0047404522000422

Bannerji, H. (2005). Building from Marx: Reflections on class and race. *Social Justice*, *32*(4), 144–160.

Baugh, J. (2018). *Linguistics in pursuit of justice.* Cambridge University Press. https://doi.org/10.1017/9781316597750

Berk-Seligson, S. (2017). *The bilingual courtroom: Court interpreters in the judicial process.* University of Chicago Press.

Billig, M. (1995). *Banal nationalism.* Sage.

Bischoff, A. (2020). The evolution of a healthcare interpreting service mapped against the bilingual health communication model: A historical qualitative case study. *Public Health Reviews*, *41*(19), 1–25. https://doi.org/10.1186/s40985-020-00123-8

Blackledge, A. (2000). Monolingual ideologies in multilingual states: Language, hegemony and social justice in Western liberal democracies. *Estudios de Sociolingüística*, *1*(2), 25–45.

Blackledge, A. (2006). The magical frontier between the dominant and the dominated: Sociolinguistics and social justice in a multilingual world. *Journal*

of Multilingual and Multicultural Development, *27*(1), 22–41. https://doi.org/10.1080/17447140608668536
Blommaert, J. (2009). Language, asylum, and the national order. *Current Anthropology*, *50*(4), 415–441.
Bourdieu, P. (1977a). The economics of linguistic exchanges. *Social Science Information*, *16*(6), 645–668. http://doi:10.1177/053901847701600601
Bourdieu, P. (1977b). *Outline of a theory of practice*. Cambridge University Press.
Bourdieu, P. (1979). Symbolic power. *Critique of Anthropology*, *4*(13–14), 77–85.
Bourdieu, P. (1984). *Distinction: A social critique of the judgement of taste*. Harvard University Press.
Bourdieu, P. (1990). *The logic of practice*. Polity Press.
Bourdieu, P. (1991). *Language and symbolic power*. Polity Press.
Bourdieu, P. (1993). *Sociology in question*. Sage.
Bourdieu, P., & Wacquant, L. J. D. (1992). *An invitation to reflexive sociology*. University of Chicago Press.
Cho, J. (2021a). 'That's not how we speak': Interpreting monolingual ideologies in courtrooms. *Griffith Law Review*, *30*(1), 50–70. https://doi.org/10.1080/10383441.2021.1932234
Cho, J. (2021b). *Intercultural communication in interpreting: Power and choices*. Routledge. https://doi.org/10.4324/9781003179993
Cho, J. (2024). Bilingual workers in a monolingual state: Bilingualism as a non-skill. *International Journal of Bilingual Education and Bilingualism*, *27*(3), 443–454. https://doi.org/10.1080/13670050.2023.2213374
Clyne, M. (1991). *Community languages: The Australian experience*. Cambridge University Press.
Clyne, M. (2005). *Australia's language potential*. UNSW Press.
Clyne, M. (2008). The monolingual mindset as an impediment to the development of plurilingual potential in Australia. *Sociolinguistic Studies*, *2*(3), 347–366.
Colic-Peisker, V. (2011). 'Ethnics' and 'Anglos' in the labour force: Advancing Australia fair?. *Journal of Intercultural Studies*, *32*(6), 637–654. https://doi.org/10.1080/07256868.2011.618108
Colley, H., & Guéry, F. (2015). Understanding new hybrid professions: Bourdieu, illusio and the case of public service interpreters. *Cambridge Journal of Education*, *45*(1), 113–131. https://doi.org/10.1080/0305764X.2014.991277
Collins, J. (1991). Hegemonic practice: Literacy and standard language in public education. In C. Mitchell, & K. Weiler (Eds.), *Rewriting literacy: Culture and the discourse of the other* (pp. 229–253). Bergin & Garvey.
Cook, V. (1999). Going beyond the native speaker in language teaching. *TESOL Quarterly*, *33*(2), 185–209.
Cushing, I. (2023). "Miss, can you speak English?": Raciolinguistic ideologies and language oppression in initial teacher education. *British Journal of Sociology of Education*, *44*(5), 896–911. https://doi.org/10.1080/01425692.2023.2206006
Dovchin, S. (2020). The psychological damages of linguistic racism and international students in Australia. *International Journal of Bilingual Education and Bilingualism*, *23*(7), 804–818. https://doi.org/10.1080/13670050.2020.1759504

Dryden, S., & Dovchin, S. (2024). Accentism: English LX users of migrant background in Australia. *Journal of Multilingual and Multicultural Development*, *45*(5), 1466–1478. https://doi.org/10.1080/01434632.2021.1980573
Eades, D. (2003). Participation of second language and second dialect speakers in the legal system. *Annual Review of Applied Linguistics*, *23*, 113–133. https://doi.org/10.1017/S0267190503000229
Elias, A., Mansouri, F., & Paradies, Y. (2021). *Racism in Australia today*. Palgrave Macmillan.
Ellis, E. (2006). Monolingualism: The unmarked case. *Estudios de Sociolingüística*, *7*(2), 173–196.
Ellis, E. (2008). Defining and investigating monolingualism. *Sociolinguistic Studies*, *2*(3), 311–330.
Ellis, E., Gogolin, I., & Clyne, M. (2010). The Janus face of monolingualism: A comparison of German and Australian language education policies. *Current Issues in Language Planning*, *11*(4), 439–460. https://doi.org/10.1080/14664208.2010.550544
Ellis, E. M. (2016). "I may be a native speaker but I'm not monolingual": Reimagining all teachers' linguistic identities in TESOL. *Tesol Quarterly*, *50*(3), 597–630.
Flores, N. (2023). Toward a raciolinguistic perspective on translation and interpretation. *Language in Society*, *52*(5), 893–901. https://doi.org/10.1017/S0047404523000660
Flores, N., & Rosa, J. (2015). Undoing appropriateness: Raciolinguistic ideologies and language diversity in education. *Harvard Educational Review*, *85*(2), 149–171. https://doi.org/10.17763/0017-8055.85.2.149
Ford, F. M. (2021). *Interpreting while black: A phenomenological study of the lived reality of African American Asl-English interpreters*. [Doctoral dissertation, Gallaudet University].
Forrest, J., Blair, K., & Dunn, K. (2021). Racist attitudes, out-groups and the Australian experience. *Australian Journal of Social Issues*, *56*(1), 78–93. https://doi.org/10.1002/ajs4.112
Gogolin, I. (1997). The "monolingual habitus" as the common feature in teaching in the language of the majority in different countries. *Per Linguam: A Journal of Language Learning*, *13*(2), 38–49. https://doi.org/10.5785/13-2-187
Goulden, R. R. (2022). *The 'forever migrant': An intersectional analysis of L/A workplace discrimination on the basis of race, African accent, and English language proficiency* [Honours dissertation, Bates College].
Grassby, A. J. (1984). *The tyranny of prejudice*. AE Press.
Hale, S. B., Bond, N., & Sutton, J. (2011). Interpreting accent in the courtroom. *Target. International Journal of Translation Studies*, *23*(1), 48–61. https://doi.org/10.1075/target.23.1.03hal
Hawthorne, L. (1997). The question of discrimination: Skilled migrants' access to Australian employment. *International Migration*, *35*(3), 395–420.
Heller, M. (2007). Bilingualism as ideology and practice. In M. Heller (Ed.), *Bilingualism: A social approach* (pp. 1–22). Palgrave Macmillan.
Heller, M., Pietikäinen, S., & Pujolar, J. (2018). *Critical sociolinguistic research methods: Studying language issues that matter*. Routledge.

Inghilleri, M. (2003). Habitus, field and discourse: Interpreting as a socially situated activity. *Target. International Journal of Translation Studies*, *15*(2), 243–268. https://doi.org/10.1075/target.15.2.03ing

Inghilleri, M. (2005). Mediating zones of uncertainty: Interpreter agency, the interpreting habitus and political asylum adjudication. *The Translator*, *11*(1), 69–85. https://doi.org/10.1080/13556509.2005.10799190

Ip, D., Lui, C. W., & Chui, W. H. (2007). Veiled entrapment: A study of social isolation of older Chinese migrants in Brisbane, Queensland. *Ageing & Society*, *27*(5), 719–738. https://doi.org/10.1017/S0144686X07006083

Kutlu, E. (2023). Now you see me, now you mishear me: Raciolinguistic accounts of speech perception in different English varieties. *Journal of Multilingual and Multicultural Development*, *44*(6), 511–525. https://doi.org/10.1080/01434632.2020.1835929

Leeman, J. (2018). It's all about English: The interplay of monolingual ideologies, language policies and the US Census Bureau's statistics on multilingualism. *International Journal of the Sociology of Language*, *2018*(252), 21–43. https://doi.org/10.1515/ijsl-2018-0013

Levon, E., Sharma, D., & Ilbury, C. (2022). *Speaking up: Accents and social mobility*. Sutton Trust.

Lippi-Green, R. (1994). Accent, standard language ideology, and discriminatory pretext in the courts. *Language in Society*, *23*(2), 163–198. https://doi.org/10.1017/S0047404500017826

Mason, I., & Ren, W. (2012). Power in face-to-face interpreting events. *Translation and Interpreting Studies*, *7*(2), 234–253. http://doi10.1075/tis.7.2.08mas

May, S. (2017). Language, imperialism, and the modern nation-state system: Implications for language rights. In O. Garcia, N. Flores, & M. Spotti (Eds.), *The Oxford handbook of language and society* (pp. 35–54). Oxford University Press. https://doi.org/10.1093/oxfordhb/9780190212896.013.12

Mesthrie, R., 2000. Critical sociolinguistics: Approaches to language and power. In R. Mesthrie, J. Swann, A. Deumert, & W. L., Leap (Eds.), *Introducing sociolinguistics* (pp. 316–353). Edinburgh University Press.

Milroy, L. (1999). Standard English and language ideology in Britain and the United States. In T. Bex, & R. J. Watts (Eds.), *Standard English: The widening debate* (pp. 173–206). Routledge.

Obasi, C. (2013). Race and ethnicity in sign language interpreter education, training and practice. *Race Ethnicity and Education*, *16*(1), 103–120. https://doi.org/10.1080/13613324.2012.733686

Pietikäinen, S. (2016). Critical debates: Discourse, boundaries and social change. In N. Coupland (Ed.), *Sociolinguistics. Theoretical debates* (pp. 263–281). Cambridge University Press.

Piller, I. (2015). Language ideologies. In K. Tracy, C. Ilie, & T. Sandel (Eds.), *The international encyclopedia of language and social interaction* (pp. 1–10). Wiley Blackwell.

Piller, I. (2016a). Monolingual ways of seeing multilingualism. *Journal of Multicultural Discourses*, *11*(1), 25–33. https://doi.org/10.1080/17447143.2015.1102921

Piller, I. (2016b). *Linguistic diversity and social justice: An introduction to applied sociolinguistics*. Oxford University Press.
Pokorn, N. K., & Čibej, J. (2017). Interpreting and linguistic inclusion – friends or foes? results from a field study. *The Translator*, *24*(2), 111–127. https://doi.org/10.1080/13556509.2017.1396406
Rida, A., & Milton, M. (2001). The non-joiners: Why migrant Muslim women aren't accessing English language classes. *Prospect*, *16*(1), 35–48.
Riggs, D. W., & Due, C. (2011). (Un)common ground?: English language acquisition and experiences of exclusion amongst new arrival students in South Australian primary schools. *Identities*, *18*(3), 273–290. https://doi.org/10.1080/1070289X.2011.635373
Rosa, J. (2019). *Looking like a language, sounding like a race*. Oxford University Press. https://doi.org/10.1080/01434632.2020.1835929
Rosa, J., & Flores, N. (2017). Unsettling race and language: Toward a raciolinguistic perspective. *Language in Society*, *46*(5), 621–647. https://doi.org/10.1017/S0047404517000562
Silverstein, M. (1979). Language structure and linguistic ideology. In P. R. Clyne, W. F. Hanks, & C. L. Hofbauer (Eds.), *The elements: A Parasession on linguistic units and levels* (pp. 193–248). Chicago Linguistic Society.
Singh, Rajendra (Ed.) (1996). *Towards a critical sociolinguistics*. John Benjamins.
Smith-Khan, L. (2017). Telling stories: Credibility and the representation of social actors in Australian asylum appeals. *Discourse & Society*, *28*(5), 512–534. https://doi.org/10.1177/0957926517710989
Smolicz, J. J. (1984). Is the monolingual nation-state out-of-date? A comparative study of language policies in Australia and the Philippines. *Comparative Education*, *20*(2), 265–285. https://doi.org/10.1080/0305006840200207
Tankosić, A., & Dovchin, S. (2023). (C)overt linguistic racism: Eastern-European background immigrant women in the Australian workplace. *Ethnicities*, *23*(5), 726–757. https://doi.org/10.1177/14687968211005104
Tankosić, A., Dryden, S., & Dovchin, S. (2021). The link between linguistic subordination and linguistic inferiority complexes: English as a second language migrants in Australia. *International Journal of Bilingualism*, *25*(6), 1782–1798. https://doi.org/10.1177/13670069211035561
Tollefson, J. W. (2006). Critical theory in language policy. In T. Ricento (Ed.), *An introduction to language policy: Theory and method* (pp. 42–59). Blackwell.
Urciuoli, B. (1995). Language and borders. *Annual Review of Anthropology*, *24*, 525–546. https://doi.org/10.1146/annurev.an.24.100195.002521
Van Parijs, P. (2011). *Linguistic justice for Europe and for the world*. Oxford University Press.
Whitlam Government minister Al Grassby dies. (2005, April 24). *The Sydney Morning Herald*. www.smh.com.au/national/whitlam-government-minister-al-grassby-dies-20050424-gdl6qq.html
Wiley, T. G. (1996). Language planning and language policy. In S. L. McKay, & N. H. Hornberger (Eds.), *Sociolinguistics and language teaching* (pp. 103–147). Cambridge University Press.

Wiley, T. G., & Lukes, M. (1996). English-only and standard English ideologies in the US. *Tesol Quarterly*, *30*(3), 511–535. https://doi.org/10.2307/3587696
Woolard, K. (1998). Introduction: Language ideology as a field of inquiry. In B. Schieffelin, K. Woolard, & P. Kroskrity (Eds.), *Language ideologies: Practice and theory* (pp. 3–47). Oxford University Press.

3 Societal monolingualism

3.1 English in imagined homogeneity

This section explores the processes by which English monolingualism was tied to the "myth of homogeneity" (Grassby, 1984, p. 2) through linguistic, racial and class relations within the context of Australian migration. The image of Australia as a white, English-speaking country has persisted ever since the colony began in the 18th century, yet Australia has never been a homogeneous nation. Before British settlement, the land was occupied by Indigenous Australians for thousands of years and at least 300 distinct languages with many more dialects were spoken (Simpson & Wigglesworth, 2019). The First Fleet, which invaded the Indigenous Australians in 1788 had British people as a majority group, yet there were also non-British people including black people of African heritage (Pybus, 2006). Such diversity was, however, rendered irrelevant to Australia, which was imagined and has remained a white country.

Australia's strong attachment to whiteness is well explained by "white colonial paranoia" (Hage, 2002), which refers to "a fear of loss of Europeanness or Whiteness and the lifestyle and privileges that are seen to emanate directly from them" (p. 419). Hage (2002) argues that far away from the mother country and isolated in the corner of the Asia-Pacific region, early settlers of Australia built the continent as an "isolated White British colony" (p. 421) to distinguish itself from what they saw as hostile and uncivilised others in the region. Paranoia tends to perceive a threat and white colonial paranoia identified 'the others' as a threat that could potentially corrupt desired white homogeneity. The others were "menaces and contagions" (Burke, 2001, p. 17), which early settlers had to keep away at all costs by fervently pursuing British identity and ignoring the presence of diverse groups.

Australia's pursuit of Britishness continued throughout its transition from a penal colony to a federation in 1901. This period was characterised by a focus on assimilating the Indigenous People into the core Anglo

DOI: 10.4324/9781032614854-3

cultures and simultaneously bringing English-speaking white migrants primarily from Britain. For much of the 19th century, assisted emigration was implemented to encourage British people to move to Australia by providing various benefits including free passages and loans (Jupp, 2004). Immigration was carefully and deliberately planned to keep Australia as British as possible (and failing that, as European as possible) and Australia is said to be "the product of conscious social engineering to create a particular kind of society" (Jupp, 2002, p. 4).

Amid efforts to build a British outpost in the South Seas, the gold rush (1850s–1860s) drew individuals from non-white and non-English-speaking backgrounds in significant numbers, leading to concerns about the desired social homogeneity of the colonies. In particular, the large number of Chinese arrivals sparked fear regarding the ethnic purity of the emerging nation, a fear which remained central for the next century (Jupp, 2002).

Immediately after the Federation of Australia came into being in 1901, the Immigration Restriction Act (1901–1959) which banned the migration by people of colour took effect and remained much of the period of 'White Australia'. 'White' was essentially 'British' as demonstrated by the deliberate concoction of census figures during this period. At various points, Australia was said to be 95 per cent British, yet that figure included everyone born in Australia, everyone born in the 50 countries of the British Empire and everyone naturalised in Australia (Grassby, 1984). Until 1949, full citizenship was automatically allowed only to British people and Australians were required to describe themselves as British, rather than Australian, in the Census until 1959 (Grassby, 1984). The Australian desire for homogeneity grounded in British identity is well exemplified by the following statement by John Curtin, a former Prime Minister (1941–1945). While this period marked a turning point in Australia's international relations by laying the groundwork for the strong Australia-U.S. alliance due to the pressures of World War II, the pursuit of British identity appears to be unaffected, as exemplified below:

> This country [Australia] shall remain forever the home of the descendants of those people who came here in peace in order to establish in the South Seas an outpost of the British race.
>
> (Department of Immigration and Border Protection, n.d.)

The pursuit of this homogeneous identity has significantly influenced the ways in which English has taken hold in Australia. The ideology of 'one nation, one language' became dominant in Australia amid rising nationalism during the period of national formation in the late-19th and early-20th century. This coincided with the global wave of aggressive nationalism, which sought nation building aimed at unification and modernisation. As the essence of a nation was tied to one standard language and monolingual speakers (Cook & Simpson, 2012; see also Section 2.1 and 2.2), many countries around the world strived to define a language symbolising national identity. For Australia that language was English (Clyne, 1991).

For Australia obsessed with whiteness, English was racialised and this is aptly demonstrated by the dictation test. Introduced in 1901 by the Immigration Restriction Act, the dictation test was a requirement for people who wished to migrate to Australia. The purpose of the test was to keep out 'the undesirable' with the requirement of passing a test in a language with which NESB people were not familiar. Originally, it was proposed that English be that language. The proposal was, however, turned down due to a possibility that non-white English speakers such as black Americans could pass the test (Crozet, 2008). It was also feared that a dictation test in English would disadvantage non-English-speaking white Europeans (Crozet, 2008) who were not as desirable as British people yet were perceived as a second-best option for migration to keep the nation as European as possible (see Jupp, 2002). Their lack of English was acceptable, because governments believed that migrants would learn English naturally (see Martin, 1978).

The preference for non-English-speaking, white people over English-speaking, non-white people, is aligned with a raciolinguistic logic according to which language and race are "jointly constructed as sets" (Rosa & Flores, 2017, p. 11; see also Section 2.2). The binary logic of the Australian case posits that one must be white to speak English; changing one's skin colour was impossible, but changing one's language was. The raciolinguistic perspective on English highlights English as a 'white language' which belonged exclusively to white people. This dimension of English monolingualism suggests that English served as a key vehicle to achieve social homogeneity characterised by linguistic and racial oneness for Australia.

The processes by which English monolingualism became entrenched were accompanied by the systematic subordination of other languages. Prior to the nationalist movement, although English was the most dominant language in Australia, local attitudes to European languages (e.g., German, French and Italian) were lenient. During the 19th century, for example, bilingual education in European languages at Australian primary schools was common. Even those languages were, however, banned in schools (with very few exceptions such as French), following the passing of the Education Acts between 1872 and 1880, which established English-monolingual state schools as a mainstream (Clyne, 1991).

In public spaces, NESB migrants were told to use English only (Clyne, 1991). At home, people were encouraged to speak English only due to a popular belief that bilingualism would harm children (Clyne, 1991). In politics, foreign languages were subject to political scrutiny as a danger to national security (Jordens, 1993). During both world wars, censorship regulation of ethnic media delivered in languages other than English made approval to publish conditional on the requirement that at least one quarter of the publication would be in English including the leading article (Gilson & Zubrzycki, 1967). Even newspapers approved for publication in other languages were not immune to political suspicion, and demand for full English translation was often made by politicians on security grounds (Jordens, 1993).

Restrictions on other languages impacted Australia's international relations too. As both cause and consequence, English monolingualism significantly contributed to the political isolationism of Australia within the Asia-Pacific region. Australia's efforts to distinguish itself from the others within the region led to ignorance of Asian cultures and languages, and a lack of language specialists in Asian languages significantly affected Australia's abilities to adequately prepare for World War II (Bostock, 1973). Not a single Australian diplomat was, however, trained in any Asian language in the post-war period between 1949 and 1958 (Bostock, 1973). Neither was any real attempt made to recruit Asian specialists into the federal government during this period, in the face of the prevailing attitude that ""you just don't need languages"" (Bostock, 1973, p. 51, emphasis in original).

The ignorance of Asian languages is not just linguistic but also racial. Ever since early settlement, Australia despised Asians as 'the uncivilised others'. This is demonstrated in Australian novels on Asia published during the first half of the 20th century. Asia is described as "innate savagery" (Vickers, 1988, p. 8) and posed a threat to white people. This oriental-racist view of Asia was also an expression of colonial anxiety in which Australia's Britishness was increasingly challenged in the post-war period and insecurity about the national identity heightened (Vickers, 1988). Creating a category which is inferior to 'us' works to enhance one's worthiness (see Cho, 2021), which reveals the blanket treatment of Asia as a strategy to cope with colonial anxiety.

Despite the fervent pursuit of homogeneity, NESB migrants increased rapidly in the mid-20th century. For one thing, Australia's massive efforts to bring in British people were not matched by the amount of British interest in migration to Australia. Furthermore, the Great Depression of the 1930s led to a decrease in migration and the birth rate (Ozolins, 1998). The resultant lack of population became a prominent issue following the end of World War II, which, in turn, led to a shift in Australian migration programs characterised by 'Populate or perish'. To bring more people in, assisted migration schemes were extended throughout Europe and beyond.

The best-known example of the post-war migration drive is Australia's acceptance of 170,000 Displaced Persons (DP) from Eastern Europe under the landmark 1947 agreement with the International Refugee Organisation. Between 1947 and 1970, approximately 728,400 migrants arrived in Australia, which accounted for 5.7 per cent of the total 1970 population (Official Year Book of the Commonwealth of Australia, 1971, as cited in Bostock, 1973).

To manage this increasing diversity, English was leveraged as a tool for assimilation. As a language which governed the nation in both practical and symbolic senses, the mastery of English served as a clear sign of assimilation into the Australian way of life (Murphy, 1952). NESB migrants were required to sign migration contracts stipulating mandatory acquisition of English upon arriving in Australia (Markus & Taft, 2015). To achieve total assimilation of migrants into Australian society, Australia's official Immigration Policy encouraged naturalisation for migrants, a loyal act during which migrants pledged their allegiance to the British Monarch, in English (Bostock, 1973). The absolute necessity of English was hardly questioned even among moderate supporters of assimilation such as Harold Holt, Minister for Immigration (1949–1952), who emphasised that:

> We should try to give them [NESB migrants] the best of what we have here in Australia, and take from them the best that they can bring to us from other lands ... Undoubtedly, one of the most effective ways to effect assimilation is a knowledge and use of the English language.
>
> (Nation's Forum of the Air, 1952, as cited in Markus & Taft, 2015)

As Australia strove to maintain homogeneity, other languages and their speakers were seen as threats to social integration (Bostock, 1973). The fear that Australian homogeneity might be tarnished by the foreign presence was shared widely, as exemplified by the 1956 speech delivered by the former president of the Australian Council of Trade Union:

> One of the first causes of friction we encounter is the fear that the presence of foreigners will undermine our own way of life. And Australian men and women cannot be blamed if they seek reassurances on this point. They are certainly not reassured by hearing foreign languages spoken in public places.
>
> (Lodewyckx, 1956, as cited in Bostock, 1973)

Amid an all-out effort to control diversity, other languages became markers of inferior class status. Most NESB migrants experienced low socioeconomic conditions, and many got straight into fields which required little English (e.g., construction), missing out on opportunities to learn English properly (Colic-Peisker, 2002). While the importance of English for assimilation was stressed, government support for language learning was significantly inadequate. English programs for migrants were provided but they were often poorly designed with a heavy focus on oral English only (Jordens, 1993). Children were excluded from English language teaching. Initial programs such as shipboard English classes for migrants and English education in the Migration Receptions Centres were available only to adults due to widespread beliefs that children would learn English naturally (Ozolins & Clyne, 2001). Inadequate language programs, long working hours, lack of opportunities to practise English, a generally low level of education and a lack of confidence among NESB migrants contributed to poor English language proficiency among migrants (Hearn, 1981).

Many migrants struggled to get by, yet their language needs were consistently ignored and denied by governments and institutions (Martin, 1978). Migrants who were not proficient in English needed translation and interpreting services, yet institutional responses to their communication needs were avoided as much as possible (Martin, 1978). Communication problems were rather blamed on migrants, which, in turn, led to the naturalisation of a perception of 'migrants as problems' (Martin, 1978). Under such circumstances, not being able to speak English well was equated with being migrants and their generally low social status.

As the number of migrants from diverse language backgrounds continued to increase, a Translation Unit was established within the Department of Immigration in 1960. It was, however, specifically tasked to deal with the mass of settlement documents, rather than assisting migrants to cope with day-to-day needs. Under such circumstances, interpreting was managed by any available bilingual speakers, and bilinguals available for interpreting were predominantly migrants (Ozolins, 1998). Newly arrived migrants had to rely on their countrymen for interpreting, sometimes for no cost and at other times for heavy costs (Camberis, 1976). Some Displaced Persons with English language proficiency worked as interpreters in the Migration Receptions Centres, while some institutions dealing with large numbers of NESB migrants (e.g., hospitals and welfare centres) witnessed emerging teams of interpreters consisting of bilingual staff members (Martin, 1978; Ozolins, 1998). There were, however, hardly any guidelines on how the job should be performed, still less on working conditions and professional identity (Ozolins, 2001).

In the absence of a central governing system, the practice of "bring your own interpreter" (Ozolins, 2001, p. 265) was widespread. Desperate situations faced by hospitals having to deal with a rapidly increasing number of NESB patients are illustrated by the use of taxi drivers as interpreters.

As medical emergencies and need for after-hours medical care increased, taxi drivers, many of whom were migrants, were hired by hospitals as interpreters. When taxi drivers were called for an interpreting job, they would turn on their meter and be paid for the amount of interpreting work they did at the hospital (Ozolins, 1998). As such, communication problems were managed only through makeshift, rather than organised institutional, measures.

With the cultural shift in the 1960s from assimilation to integration, language as a significant factor in the poverty experienced among NESB migrants began to emerge as a social issue (see Henderson et al., 1970; Masterman & Wentworth, 1969). Such findings, however, persistently met with government denial. In the first series of reports on migrant poverty led by Professor Ronald Henderson in 1970, the findings pointed to a lack of English as a major cause of migrant poverty but were met with defensive reactions from the Ministry of Immigration. According to the Programme Development Sub-section of the Ministry:

> The basic fallacy involved in extrapolating from the survey is that while it gives a fair picture of those poor who are migrants, it ignores those migrants who are not poor.
>
> (Planning and Development Branch, 1972, as cited in Jordens, 1993)

Amid government denial and procrastination on language problems, migrants began to leave Australia. A federal parliamentary inquiry into the increasing numbers of migrants returning to their home countries was conducted between 1967 and 1973. The results revealed language and communication as the most significant factor behind the increasing departures (Jordens, 1993).

Despite the increasing evidence on communication as a cause of migrant struggles, it was not until 1973 that the national government began to act. The Immigration Department's *Report on the Survey of Interpreting and Translating Needs in the Community* was published that year (Jordens, 1993). The study, based on responses to 2,515 questionnaires sent to 34 different types of organisations in areas with a large migrant population, flagged inadequate language services as the main culprit behind migrants' failure to access essential services to which they were entitled and to manage daily life within the boundaries of laws (Jordens, 1993). Embarrassed by the findings, the government finally acknowledged communication problems as a leading cause of migrant struggles and took action by looking into the possibility of formal provision of translation and interpreting. It is against this backdrop of the blind pursuit of social homogeneity, entrenched English monolingualism tied to race and class, and persistent denial of communication problems that translation and interpreting began in Australia.

3.2 The beginning of interpreting

The early-1970s, during which translation and interpreting was first introduced, were a time of changing political conditions characterised by the transition from White Australia to multiculturalism. By the 1960s, the White Australia policy became increasingly untenable due to mounting domestic pressures and increasing international criticism. This was accompanied by growing awareness of linguistic and cultural diversity and institutional responsibilities for communication with NESB migrants in essential areas including education, industrial relations, welfare and public administration (Martin, 1978; Ozolins, 1998). At the same time, ethnic groups and local activists began to lobby for policies targeting migrant inequalities, specifically demanding the establishment of translation and interpreting services (Hlavac, 2016).

Communication as a cause of inequity was evident in the disproportionate number of work injuries and invalidism among NESB migrants. Many migrants were forced to undertake work of a lower standard than their previous jobs at home due to the difficulties with recognition of their overseas qualifications by Australian authorities (Hearn, 1981). Unskilled migrants got into any jobs that were available (Krupinski, 1984) and became significantly overrepresented in low-skilled occupations, which were prone to work injuries (Bollini & Siem, 1995). As NESB migrants were unable to follow safety instructions in English, many ended up getting injured and were significantly overrepresented in workers' compensation litigation cases (Bollini & Siem, 1995). Those who were injured were doubly disadvantaged due to communication issues with authorities, which made little attempt to take responsibility to ensure proper communication with NESB migrants. According to the 1977 Commission of Inquiry into Poverty:

> ... [many migrants] are turned away or give up as they are passed from one agency to another in their endeavour to find someone with whom they can communicate.
>
> (quoted in Byrnes, 1979, p. 14)

Against this backdrop, a series of major developments regarding translation and interpreting took place. In 1973, the free Emergency Telephone Interpreter Service was introduced as a world first. Referred to as "one of the most remarkable innovations of Australian language policy" (Ozolins, 2001, p. 259), the 24-hour service of telephone interpreting was introduced at first to Sydney and Melbourne, where the most disadvantaged groups of migrants were concentrated. Many migrants chose those cities as initial residences because it was relatively easy to find jobs and cheaper accommodation there (Byrnes, 1979). Telephone interpreting was designed to address issues arising from local areas in which communication challenges were compounded by distance and a scattered population (Department of Immigration, 1973). As the popularity of the service increased, it became the Telephone Interpreting Service (TIS), covering not just emergency but also other day-to-day communication needs.

The establishment of telephone interpreting, however, did not address fundamental issues including the disorganisation and quality of language services. A series of government initiatives in the early 1970s led to an awakening to the need for formalisation of translation and interpreting to improve quality and standards. In 1974, a report entitled *Language Barrier* was published by the Working Party on Interpreters set up by the Committee on Overseas Professional Qualifications to determine the range of tasks which needed language service provision. The report also identified problems including non-systematic operation of translation and interpreting, institutional under-recognition of the need for interpreters and potential impact of non-provision of language services on NESB migrants. For example:

> ... experience to date appears to suggest that employers will tend to underrate the level of interpreter required just as they have, over the past twenty-five years, underrated the need for interpreters of any kind. In both cases this may lead to the violation of the human and civil rights of those involved.
>
> (quoted in Byrnes, 1979, p. 83)

The report also discovered the lack of quality interpreting services nationwide was one of the most significant issues (Hearn, 1981). In order to professionalise translation and interpreting, the National Accreditation Authority for Translators and Interpreters (NAATI) was instituted in 1977 by the government. NAATI introduced an accreditation scheme for both translation and interpreting and made it mandatory for anyone who wished to work as a translator and/or interpreter in Australia to pass the exam. The interpreting accreditation system categorised professional competence into five specific levels, ranging from the lowest level of bilingual aides (bilingual public servants who use their bilingual skills for work) to the most advanced level of senior advanced interpreters capable of managing conference interpreting (Ozolins, 2001). NAATI also worked with the Migrant Education Review Committee of the Commonwealth Education Department to support the development of interpreter services by setting educational standards, developing courses and setting up organisational infrastructure relevant to interpreting (Hearn, 1981).

The formal establishment of NAATI is said to mark a shift in the government's perception of multilingualism from a liability to a recognised principle of access and equity for all (Hlavac, 2016). Moving away from Anglo-centrism, multicultural Australia officially recognised linguistic diversity, finally accepting other languages which had long been ignored (Clyne, 1991; Ozolins, 1985).

In line with this cultural shift, translation and interpreting became a central focus in a series of major government policies. To begin with, the 1978 Galbally review of migrant programs and services drew specific attention to a lack of proper English language education catering to migrants who came with different levels of education. According to the report, 400,000 adult migrants arrived from non-English-speaking countries between 1967/8 and 1976/7, yet only 21,035 people attended full-time English language courses. Defining Australia as a country where "all members of our society must have equal opportunity to realise their full potential and must have equal access to programs and services" (Galbally, 1978, p. 4), the report specifically recommended the establishment of language specialist services for the areas of health care, education and law.

Translation and interpreting emerged as a key area of national language policy as well. The early 1980s saw a strong political interest in embracing a diverse range of ethnic, language and language professional groups in language policies. In 1982, a Senate inquiry into language policy in Australia was carried out, producing the *Report on a National Language Policy* in 1984. It identified a considerable number of issues that needed to be addressed in a national language policy and presented the following four guiding principles for a policy:

1. Competence in English
2. Maintenance and development of languages other than English
3. Provision of services in languages other than English
4. Opportunities for learning second languages

The third pillar, "provision of services in languages other than English", of which translation and interpreting forms a significant part, illustrates growing political recognition of language services for Australia's diverse population (Ozolins, 2001). Along these four main pillars, Lo Bianco (1987) published the *National Policy on Languages* (NPL), the first comprehensive language policy in Australia. The goal of "provision of services in languages other than English" in the NPL presented translation and interpreting as the vanguards of multilingualism and multiculturalism in order to actualise cultural and educational enrichment, economic benefits and enhanced national standing in the region and beyond.

Translation and interpreting continued to receive policy attention throughout the 1980s and 1990s concurrently with Australia's increasing engagement with Asia and the rising importance of Asian languages. The National Asian Languages and Studies in Australian Schools (NALSAS) Strategy (1996–2002) is a prominent example to illustrate this shift. Focusing on four Asian languages – Chinese, Indonesian, Japanese and Korean – the NALSAS strategy specifically recommended that the government provide funding to support both Asian language learning and Asian studies more broadly. For the former, the strategy set the target participation rate of 25% for languages at Year 12 level, recommending that 15% of students study one of the designated languages. The strategy is distinguished from other similar policies due to the establishment of qualitative targets for which interpreting was specifically set as the highest level of language proficiency. For example:

> A narrow group of highly proficient graduates capable of becoming (with further training) future interpreters with native-level fluency, a larger group of prospective university graduates capable of developing the Year 12 proficiency outcomes to the degree that their languages/cultures skills are of direct professional relevance to the university disciplines they pursue (e.g. engineering graduates with professionally useful Indonesian, Japanese speaking lawyers, Chinese speaking commerce graduates) to a much broader group again capable of servicing requirements, say, of Australian services industries (e.g. tourism) in sales positions where some level of proficiency would be useful in dealing with clients.
>
> (Council of Australian Governments, 1994, p. xi, as cited in Liddicoat, 2009)

This series of engagements with translation and interpreting in language policy illustrates that translation and interpreting, literally invisible two decades ago, came to claim a legitimate place in the political domain. At the same time, however, it is important to question whether the official recognition of translation and interpreting was accompanied by increased public recognition of linguistic diversity and communication problems experienced by migrants. Asking this is particularly relevant considering the long-standing domination of English, disregard for other languages and their speakers, and the tendency to deny communication problems in Australia.

The examination of the question reveals a gap between the official recognition of linguistic diversity and public awareness. Throughout the 1970s, significant progress was achieved in the promotion of linguistic diversity following the multicultural turn. In addition to the institutionalisation of translation and interpreting, state multilingual broadcasting stations (e.g., SBS) were established to ensure ethnic rights to languages. In education, 25 languages were introduced to the Matriculation Examinations. General awareness of languages, was however, much slower, developing only very gradually (Clyne, 1988). In 1978, a year after NAATI was established, the attitudes to language learning remained extremely narrow even among Australian intellectuals and language experts. For example:

> [languages other than English are] essentially unlearnable by normal people, and ... Australians have a special innate anti-talent for learning them while English is learnable ... by speakers of other languages. (Submission from the Australian Linguistic Society to the Prime Minister, October 1978, as citied in Clyne, 2004).
>
> ... there is no possibility at all that most Anglo-Australians will become bilingual in English and any other language, let alone in one of the ethnic languages. Nor is there the slightest reason to give such linguistic proficiency a high educational priority.
>
> (Partington, 1981, p. 472)

This expressed inability to understand the workings and values of language learning among intellectuals suggests that language awareness in the public might have been even poorer. Bilingualism continued to be under-appreciated across society especially in universities where language learning was largely treated irrelevant and unnecessary (Bostock, 1973). While Australia was officially declared a multicultural nation, the country was still the land of monoglots (Kerr, 1981). Social prejudice against foreign speech and their speakers remained strong (West, 1980). After all, it was a country where the attitude that "you just don't need languages" had prevailed for so long. How would it have been possible for such attitudes to change dramatically without massive government efforts to promote public awareness of linguistic diversity?

The mismatch between the multicultural emphasis on diversity and the continued hostility to other languages and speakers was also attributable to the inadequate consideration of key social issues in the process of introducing multiculturalism. While multiculturalism itself represents significant policy progress, it was a reactive, rather than a proactive, response to the White Australia policy, which was dismantled under mounting pressure (Ang, 2005). In a rush to introduce multiculturalism to end White Australia, the government failed to properly consider and address important social issues from the previous era: language was one of them (Smolicz, 1984). The issue of race did not receive attention either, for racial hierarchies were treated as irrelevant in multicultural Australia (Ang, 2005).

The mismatch between the ideal and practice of language services is illustrated by the significant underuse of translation and interpreting in government institutions. Despite the free provision of language services, the old practice of bringing your own interpreter was prevalent (Jupp, 2004). Another public, dominant attitude to translation and interpreting was that language service provision would only discourage migrants from learning English (Hearn, 1981). For one thing, NAATI did not have the power to make language service provision mandatory (Ozolins, 2001). As interpreter use was entirely at the user's discretion, individual awareness of linguistic diversity and communication problems mattered significantly.

Considering inadequate awareness of language and continued English monolingualism, it is natural to ask how the emerging profession of interpreting navigated the entrenched English monolingualism and prejudice against other languages and speakers. The next section examines this question by focusing on health care interpreting, an emerging bilingual profession in the "most monolingual industrialized nation in the world" (Bostock, 1978).

3.3 Unrecognised profession

In 1977, the NSW Health Care Interpreter Service was launched as the first of its kind in Australia, covering interpreters in all major health institutions. It was followed by the establishment of interpreting services under the Department of Education of Victoria, which dealt with not only education-related matters but also health issues of NESB students (e.g., counselling). Both services focused on high-demand languages such as Arabic, Greek, Italian, Serbian and Croatian, Spanish and Turkish. Asian languages (e.g., Chinese, Vietnamese, Cambodian and Laotian) were added a year later in 1978.

Around the time of the launch of the interpreter services, Australian health care remained fundamentally monolingual and monocultural. Since inception, health care institutions in Australia had been dominated by Anglo-Celtic Australians, a structure normalised within the racialised social hierarchy (Shoebridge, 1980). Just as discrimination and inequality against minority groups were naturalised in the society, inequity was deeply ingrained in Australian health care. This is exemplified by the prevalence of racism against Indigenous populations, a problem which is still present in contemporary Australia (Durey, 2015). Whilst problematic, discrimination may not always be a conscious practice but an outcome of a combination of both conscious and unconscious behaviours.

The latter means that members of the privileged group do not recognise their behaviours as discriminatory in an environment in which relations of dominance were accepted as common sense (Durey, 2015; see also Bourdieu & Wacquant, 2002).

English-speaking Anglo health care providers dominated the system, with migrants located at the bottom of the hierarchy as cleaners and kitchen staff (Shoebridge, 1980). Even after the introduction of the multicultural policy, there was little understanding of migrant health issues as problems relating to social structures. In line with the prevailing public view of 'migrants as problems' (Martin, 1978), health care institutions regarded NESB migrants as a nuisance, a perception which was exacerbated within the hierarchical power structures (Shoebridge, 1980). In a form of elite knowledge production, unsubstantiated opinions and stereotyping ideas produced by white doctors regarding NESB migrants were widely circulated within the health care sector (Shoebridge, 1980). For example, back injuries were common in heavy labour, yet the injuries were defined as ethnic, rather than medical, problems depending on the most dominant ethnic group in the industry (Grassby, 1984). With expressions such as 'Irish back', 'Italian back' and 'Lebanese back' common, the dominant attitude was that if you were different and had a bad back, then it was an ethnic problem, not a medical one (Grassby, 1984).

Perhaps not surprisingly, there was little awareness of communication problems as an institutional responsibility. Many medical staff who were monolinguals in English regarded communication as non-critical to diagnoses of NESB patients (Shoebridge, 1980). Taking non-English-speaking mental patients as an example, when those suspected of having mental illnesses were reported by camp managers or employment officers to hospitals, doctors made a diagnosis based on what other people able to speak English, no matter how little, alleged that the patients had said and done, rather than trying to communicate properly with patients (Murphy, 1952). Hospitals often relied on migrant staff such as kitchen workers to deal with delicate negotiations concerning life and surgery (Grassby, 1984). In desperate situations, medical staff depended on "anyone who was even slightly bilingual" (Hearn, 1981, p. 19) including both the willing and the unwilling, even cleaners, clerks, children and other patients. For certain medical conditions which required extreme precision for treatment, this communication practice meant the difference between life and death; inability to communicate led to tragedy in some cases (Hearn, 1981).

It is within this context of institutional monolingualism, inadequate awareness of communication problems and power hierarchies that the health care interpreter services began.

In a rare study based on interviews with pioneer health care interpreters in New South Wales and Victoria, Hearn (1981) identified four main problems reported by the first interpreters: the value of the services; professional acceptance; uncertainty about continuity; and conditions of work. It is important to note how problems experienced by the interpreters related to biases against migrants including interpreters.

As for the first point regarding the value of the interpreting services, the participants expressed strong beliefs in the importance of their work for NESB populations, taking pride in the differences they could make for the marginalised. The work itself was reported to be demanding, yet the participants were motivated by a sense of humanity and positive change they brought to the institutional processes. At the same time, however, the participants expressed frustration at the institutional lack of understanding about the nature of language barriers. Even with interpreter assistance, NESB migrants often experienced difficulties expressing themselves clearly due to feeling intimidated in a strange environment. Furthermore, most NESB migrants had little education and sometimes lacked confidence expressing their ideas clearly. Health care providers who were predominantly from English-speaking, Anglo backgrounds failed to understand the challenges experienced by NESB patients and tended to see patients as problems. For example:

> I don't think many Australians realise just how difficult, I would say frightening, it is to be a migrant, unable to communicate in a strange environment.
>
> (p. 51)

> Many of them [migrants] have a low level of education and feel inferior in the presence of educated people.
>
> (p. 50)

The lack of language awareness among health care providers relates to the second point, professional acceptance. The study points out general attitudes to interpreting as non-essential and deliberate avoidance of using interpreters among health care providers. A general tendency was reported, which viewed interpreting as a semi-profession among established professionals (e.g., doctors, nurses and psychologists). Those professionals treated interpreters as assistants or helpers who were inferior in the established professional hierarchy. For example:

> His [doctor's] response was: "They (the interpreters) are here to do what we say, not to tell us what to do". Even though I know the doctor was at fault, he made me feel inferior and helpless.
>
> (p. 54)

While the precarious employment status of interpreters who were lowly paid and under-supported is identified as one factor behind such rejection, it was also health care providers' fear of losing power that contributed to the under-recognition of interpreting. That is, providers who enjoyed absolute power for many years saw interpreters as intruders into their entrenched domain of professional dominance (Shoebridge, 1980). For health care providers who were used to exercising sole power over medical decisions, reliance on interpreters was tantamount to losing their exclusive privilege (Shoebridge, 1980).

Another important factor behind the problem of acceptance was racial and class biases. All of the early interpreters were migrants, a natural outcome of mass migration, English monolingualism and ignorance of other languages. The concentration of migrants in interpreting, however, was seen less favourably due to the social hierarchies in which NESB migrants were predominantly regarded as a "'second class citizenship'" (Hearn, 1981, p. 7, emphasis in original). The migrant aspect of interpreting was further accentuated by the fact that people served by interpreters were also migrants who were perceived as ignorant and deficient. The persistent perception of interpreting was that it was an unnecessary service for migrants who should be learning English, rather than depending on interpreters. For example:

> They believe we are providing a special service for migrants at their expense. They see us as a form of discrimination in favour of migrants. (p. 56)

The lack of acceptance and professional respect was further compounded by the final two points of uncertainty about continuity and conditions of work. At the time of the interviews, the participants were struggling under the "twin evils of institutional uncertainty and what might be termed "'professional identity crisis'" (p. 61, emphasis in original). The report found that job insecurity prevailed among the participants. As the first-ever major scheme for NESB migrants, the health care interpreting services were still on trial and were constantly under review and threats of budget reductions. Under such pressures, interpreters' working conditions including remuneration, leave entitlement and clear career structures were not given sufficient consideration (Byrnes, 1979). This further contributed to the lack of professional respect among health care providers who treated interpreters as temporary workers, assistants and machines (Byrnes, 1979). Frustrations felt by the interpreters about job uncertainties and unrecognition are demonstrated by the following excerpts:

> I felt quite embarrassed almost as if I had to justify my presence.
>
> (p. 59)

> They [health care providers] also try to make it clear to the patients that we are not equals.
>
> (p. 63)

> A lot of them seem to think we are lucky to have a job.
>
> (p. 64)

At the end of the interviews, the participants were asked about what needed to be done to improve interpreting services. They responded by emphasising the need for health care providers and institutions to be educated and trained in working with interpreters and NESB patients. The recommendations made by the interpreters include:

- Training of health care professionals regarding cultural sensitivity of NESB patients
- Awareness-raising among health care professionals regarding the importance of interpreting
- Improvement of publicity and public education regarding the necessity for interpreting services
- More engagement of interpreters in health care interactions as co-professionals
- Removal of racial biases against interpreters and interpreting services as special schemes for migrants
- An increase in the number of health care interpreters
- Training for interpreters regarding medical expertise and interaction handling

The experiences of the first cohort of health care interpreters highlight interpreting as an unrecognised profession in a monolingual health care milieu. In an environment in which linguistic, racial and class prejudices were deeply entrenched, interpreting was devalued, with interpreters subject to mistreatment by health care professionals in superior positions. Under such circumstances, both interpreters and NESB patients whom they served were seen as problems. Shoebridge (1980) further exemplifies this point with the 1980 Conference on Ethnic and Immigration Studies, held several years after the introduction of multiculturalism. Although it purported to focus on migrants in health care, the conference nevertheless approached migrants from Anglo-centric perspectives. These saw NESB migrants and their culture as deficient, emphasising strong needs to educate ignorant migrants about the Australian health care system. Similarly, health care interpreters were regarded as inadequate yet without solid evidence; it was recommended they be trained to be more adequate for purpose. While education for migrants and interpreters was strongly recommended, no mention was made of the need for health care providers to make corresponding efforts to understand other languages and cultures.

The findings provide an important glimpse into how the linguistic, racial and class hierarchies were so deeply entrenched in the monolingual environment of Australian health care that they continued to influence the ways in which interpreting was perceived and treated. They also illuminate how institutional monolingualism and prejudices against other languages and speakers set the tone for the profession of interpreting as a rewarding yet ignored profession.

3.4 Continued problems

Throughout the 1980s and 1990s, translation and interpreting expanded significantly to meet an increasing number of NESB migrants. Asian languages which had been unavailable for NAATI testing were included in NAATI accreditation process. Indigenous languages and Australian Sign Language (Auslan) interpreting were also included for NAATI accreditation in line with the growing recognition of the rights of Indigenous populations and deaf people (Hlavac, 2021). And a private language service market grew, focusing primarily on medico-legal and legal work (Ozolins, 1998). As the private market developed, the number of interpreters working in it also increased.

Health care interpreting expanded too, as exemplified by the establishment of the Central Health Interpreter Service in Victoria in 1982, which was followed by similar provisions across all states in Australia. The Victorian service is noteworthy for improved benefits such as paid travel time for interpreters (Hlavac, 2021). Another key development was the establishment of migrant health units in many states, beginning in 1984. These units were tasked with dealing with four types of problems: language barriers, lack of information and unequal access to services, culturally inappropriate services and prejudices, and inadequate involvement of ethnic groups in health services improvement (Chu, 1998). As migrant health gained institutional status, it gave a boost to interpreter employment. Overall, remuneration was relatively high and full-time employment of interpreters was substantial (Hlavac, 2021). The establishment of the Australian Institute of Interpreters and Translators (AUSIT) in 1987 as the professional association of language service providers also marked an important milestone for translation and interpreting in Australia.

While interpreting as a profession was being established in Australia, perception, however, remained a problem. Interpreters continued to struggle in terms of professional identity due to a lack of professional respect and lower occupational status. The work was hardly regarded as professional work and was often seen as something that could easily be replaced by any bilinguals such as English-speaking family members and friends (Ozolins, 1998). Interpreters continued to be identified with the migrant clients they served, rather than being acknowledged as language experts in their own right (Ozolins, 1998). Some health care interpreters performed their roles as interpreters, yet others did jobs other than interpreting, more as general hospital workers, with the continued perception of interpreters as someone who speaks more than one language rather than a skilled language worker (Ozolins, 1998).

The poor perception of interpreting further deteriorated with changes in government approaches to language provision services. Beginning in the late 1980s, conservative politics dominated the Australian political scene, along with the re-emergence of racist debates led, most prominently, by the One Nation Party. Furthermore, a neoliberal turn of major global politics influenced Australia, prioritising efficiency and streamlining. This led to reform drives in Australian health care characterised by massive restructuring, downsizing of public hospitals and severe funding cuts in migrant health units (Chu, 1998). As health care budgets tightened, interpreter services were significantly affected (Garrette et al., 2009). Language work began to be contracted out by public sector agencies, and a range of expenses previously covered by the employers (e.g., travel costs) had to be borne by language workers themselves (Association of Professional Engineers, Scientists and Managers, 2012; Translators and Interpreters Australia, 2020). This, in turn, led most interpreters to work as freelancers for profit-seeking private language service providers (Hlavac, 2021).

While the health care interpreting services survived the changes, the perception of interpreting remained extremely poor. A rare study on problems with the use of health care interpreting services in 1997, twenty years after the launch of the health care interpreter service, reveals that little progress had been achieved in terms of institutional awareness of interpreting. Blackford et al. (1997) identify the following major problems relating to health care interpreting use:

- Health care providers not knowing how to work with interpreters
- Insufficient training of health care providers on the use of interpreter services
- Subjective and arbitrary decisions on the use of interpreters among health care providers

- Unsystematic ways of assessing NESB patients' English language proficiency
- Disengagement between admission clerks and health care providers regarding language needs of NESB patients
- Nurses' disengagement with interpreting services
- Insufficient time allocated to interpreter-mediated medical consultations which required at least double the standard consultation time
- Incompatibility between hospitals' inpatient computer systems and the centralised interpreter booking system used by the Medical Records Department, preventing information exchange regarding patients' language needs

The identified issues may appear to be systemic problems yet are essentially perception problems. Nurses operated as gatekeepers with strong control over patient access to interpreting and their awareness of linguistic diversity and interpreting was, therefore, critical to ensure access equity. Despite such importance, the study found that nursing staff had never considered communication problems as part of nursing practice, seeing those problems as exclusively belonging to NESB patients. Even if NESB patients successfully managed to arrange interpreters, health care providers who had never been trained in working with interpreters did not know how to work with them. Despite recommendations for allocating more time for interpreter-mediated consultations by some states (e.g., Health Department Victoria), most hospitals ignored such recommendations. Perhaps not surprisingly, management of communication problems was regarded as the interpreter's own responsibility, rather than collaborative work with health care providers.

The poor perception of interpreting has, indeed, significantly undermined the development of the profession. Officially, health care interpreting has been recognised in both social and health policies for its importance to ensure access equity and health outcomes for linguistic minorities (Hlavac et al., 2018). In practice, however, interpreting has hardly been regarded as a legitimate profession. A close look at *In Touch*, a quarterly translation and interpreting magazine published by AUSIT, reveals the perception of the profession as chronic. Unlike other professions, translation and interpreting qualifications have been deemed inessential for recruitment of language workers; anyone who claims to be bilingual is generally hired for translation and interpreting work (Bouassi, 2014). This has allowed many untrained bilinguals to enter the market, a situation exacerbated by private language service providers keen to maximise profits by using cheap labour (Hirmiz, 2014; see also Section 4.3.2).

Analysis of *In Touch* also identifies that the image of language services was often tarnished by their very nature as welfare services (Ozolins, 2016). The public sector, which was the biggest client of language services tended to associate language services with "'poor bugger who doesn't speak English'" (Ozolins, 2016, p. 11, emphasis in original). This perception of translation and interpreting as welfare services for poor migrants affected not only its reputation but also the resources essential to the development of language services (Ozolins, 2016).

The continued inadequate perception of interpreting is well demonstrated by the significant under-utilisation of health care interpreting in Australian hospitals. In 2000, the Doctors' Priority Line was established to effectively remove language barriers by enabling speedy access to interpreters for doctors. Under the system, which runs 24 hours a day for seven days a week, doctors can generally access interpreters within three minutes of a call, for free. Despite the availability of free interpreter services, however, as few as 1% of General Practitioner (GP) consultations for patients with limited English were previously reported to routinely engage professional interpreter services (Phillips & Travaglia, 2011; Schulz, 2020; Vanstone et al., 2013). Interpreter engagement in Australian health care, indeed, remains significantly substandard to date (Migrant & Refugee Health Partnership, 2020). Bilingual communication is commonly managed by *ad hoc* interpreters or individuals who are not trained for interpreting, despite the high risks associated with communication errors and negative health outcomes for patients with limited proficiency in the dominant language (Saito et al., 2021; White et al., 2018).

Research on the under-use of health care interpreting generally views the low uptake of interpreting as systemic issues including time constraints of doctors, booking complexities, budgets, health care providers' lack of knowledge about interpreting and interpreter shortages (Chang et al., 2021; Kerrigan et al., 2021). While clearly relevant, the clinical approaches focus on problems *within* the systems, overlooking Australia's broader social milieu, in which interpreting has been significantly under-recognised in relation to linguistic, racial and class biases. Ignorance of interpreting is essentially ignorance of minority groups who have no other means but to rely on interpreting to communicate their health needs. It is also essentially an issue of social justice and human rights, considering the high risk posed by miscommunication of health information for NESB patients (see Al Shamsi et al., 2020; Flores et al., 2012; Showstack, 2019). The examination of the processes by which health care interpreting has developed in Australia reveals strong ties between monolingualism and the under-recognition of interpreting, with general perception of interpreting as one significant area needing improvement.

3.5 Summary

This chapter has examined how English monolingualism has been entrenched at the intersections between language, race and class within the migration context of Australia. It has also explored how entrenched English monolingualism has influenced the development of health care interpreting, identifying the ties between English monolingualism and the poor perception of interpreting. By paying attention to the ties between the local sociolinguistic conditions and interpreting, the chapter has demonstrated that social attitudes to other languages and speakers impact interpreting as a profession and practice. The chapter identifies four important findings.

First, the historical examination of English monolingualism in Australia reveals monolingualism as not only linguistic but also a racialised and class-based practice within the specific context of Australia. As amply discussed, the colonial anxiety relating to geographical isolation led Australia to fervently pursue social homogeneity. The pursuit of homogeneity was further strengthened during White Australia, which represented an unprecedented social engineering project in modern history. As the language of the U.K., the mother land, English became strongly tied to the homogeneous identity characterised by Britishness and whiteness. English represented a white language, which was imagined to belong exclusively to white people, as exemplified in the case of the dictation test. English was also used to keep social unity by homogenising language among NESB migrants. It was a marker of social class too, because migrants were often not fluent in English and ended up in poverty. The findings highlight English as a key tool for social unity and homogeneity within the unique sociolinguistic conditions of Australia.

Second, the chapter highlights the strong ties between interpreting and the specific sociolinguistic conditions of Australia. As illustrated, English monolingualism caused a great deal of suffering for NESB migrants, yet government responsibilities for addressing communication problems for linguistic minorities were avoided as much as possible. With governments in denial of communication problems experienced by migrants, people not fluent in English were framed as problems, which, in turn, strengthened biases against other languages and speakers. Born out of the tensions between the ideal of social homogeneity and the reality of increasing diversity, interpreting represents an ideological site in which the intricacies of linguistic, racial and class interactions can be best observed.

Third, the findings illuminate the linguistic, racial and class biases as primary culprits behind the under-recognition of interpreting. While the formalisation of language service provision was an important step in delivering equity for all, the entrenched English monolingualism impacted the ways in which interpreting was perceived and practised. As exemplified in the case of the first health care interpreting services, interpreting was predominantly seen as a welfare service provided by migrants for migrants.

With NESB migrants seen as a problem and second-class citizens, working for this stigmatised group impacted the general perception of interpreting as low in professional and social hierarchies. The unfavourable perception of interpreting was exacerbated in the English-monolingual, Anglo-centric health care sector, which regarded interpreters as different and a necessary evil. The findings provide an important glimpse into the key question of this book, which is why interpreting is under-appreciated in Australia, despite its criticality for access equity and social inclusion.

Fourth, the findings reveal a big gap between the interpreting system and the perception of interpreting. In the English-speaking Anglophone world, Australia is the only country which provides free health care interpreting services and is regarded internationally as a model of interpreting service provision (Phillips & Travaglia, 2011). While Australia has made considerable efforts to promote access equity through the formalisation and provision of language services, the analysis set out in this chapter illustrates a lack of awareness and understanding of interpreting among health care institutions and providers as a persistent problem. The old perception of 'any bilingual can interpret' has continued, as exemplified by the common use of bilingual family members, and interpreters are found to have struggled with the issue of professional legitimacy all along. The lack of appreciation for interpreting closely relates to the institutional monolingual milieu which is situated in broader societal monolingualism.

Taken together, the findings highlight the under-appreciation of interpreting as a problem deeply embedded in historical monolingual biases relating to language, race and class. It emphasises inadequate perception of interpreting as one significant problem which has impacted the development of health care interpreting. The chapter shows that the problem of the under-appreciation of interpreting is not just an occupational issue, but a social issue deeply implicated in linguistic, racial and class hierarchies.

References

Al Shamsi, H., Almutairi, A. G., Al Mashrafi, S., & Kalbani, T. A. (2020). Implications of language barriers for healthcare: A systematic review. *Oman Medical Journal*, *35*(2), 1–7. https://doi.org/10.5001/omj.2020.40

Ang, I. (2005). *On not speaking Chinese: Living between Asia and the West*. Routledge.

Association of Professional Engineers, Scientists and Managers. (2012). *Lost in translation. Barriers to building a sustainable Australian translating and interpreting industry*. APESMA.

Blackford, J., Street, A., & Parsons, C. (1997). Breaking down language barriers in clinical practice. *Contemporary Nurse*, 6(1), 15–21. https://doi.org/10.5172/conu.1997.6.1.15

Bollini, P., & Siem, H. (1995). No real progress towards equity: Health of migrants and ethnic minorities on the eve of the year 2000. *Social Science & Medicine*, *41*(6), 819–828. https://doi.org/10.1016/0277-9536(94)00386-8

Bostock, W. (1973). Monolingualism in Australia. *The Australian Quarterly*, *45*(2), 39–52. https://doi.org/10.2307/20634564

Bostock, W. W. (1978). On elections, voting and participation: The linguistic and cultural prerequisites for participation in Australian society. *Politics*, *13*(1), 155–158. https://doi.org/10.1080/00323267808401649

Bouassi, T. (2014). Interpreters deserve better recognition for their training and qualifications. *In Touch*, *22*(3), 6.

Bourdieu, P., & Wacquant, L. (2002) *An invitation to reflexive sociology*. Polity Press.

Burke, A. (2001). *In fear of security: Australia's invasion anxiety*. Pluto Press.

Byrnes, S. J. (1979). An evaluation of the health care interpreter service of the inner metropolitan region of the health commission of New South Wales [Doctoral dissertation, UNSW Sydney].

Camberis, M. (1976). Problems of ethnic groups in our community. *Australian Journal of Physiotherapy*, *22*(1), 42–46.

Chang, H., Hutchinson, C., & Gullick, J. (2021). Pulled away: The experience of bilingual nurses as ad hoc interpreters in the emergency department. *Ethnicity & Health*, *26*(7), 1045–1064. https://doi.org/10.1080/13557858.2019.1613518

Cho, J. (2021). Constructing a white mask through English: The misrecognized self in Orientalism. *International Journal of the Sociology of Language*, *2021*(271), 17–34. https://doi.org/10.1515/ijsl-2020-0037

Chu, C. (1998). Cross-cultural health issues in contemporary Australia. *Ethnicity & Health*, *3*(1–2), 125–134. https://doi.org/10.1080/13557858.1998.9961854

Clyne, M. (1988). Australia's national policy on languages and its implications. *Journal of Education Policy*, *3*(3), 273–280. https://doi.org/10.1080/02680 93880030306

Clyne, M. (1991). *Community languages: The Australian experience*. Cambridge University Press.

Clyne, M. (2004). Trapped in a monolingual mindset. *Principal Matters*, *59*, 18–20.

Colic-Peisker, V. (2002). Croatians in Western Australia: Migration, language and class. *Journal of Sociology*, *38*(2), 149–166.

Cooke, M., & Simpson, J. (2012). Discourses about linguistic diversity. In A. Blackledge, A. Creese & M. Martin-Jones (Eds.), *The Routledge handbook of multilingualism* (pp. 116–130). Routledge.

Crozet, C. (2008). Australia's linguistic culture and its impact on languages education. *Babel*, *42*(3), 19–24.

Department of Immigration. (1973). *Report on the Survey of Interpreting and Translating Needs in the Community*. https://nla.gov.au/nla.obj-1746204121/ view?partId=nla.obj-1751649758

Department of Immigration and Border Protection. (n.d.). *Fact Sheet – Abolition of the 'White Australia' Policy*. www.border.gov.au/about/ corporate/information/factsheets/08abolition

Durey, A. (2015). Antonio Gramsci and Pierre Bourdieu: 'Whiteness' and indigenous healthcare. In Collyer, F. (Ed.), *The Palgrave handbook of social theory in health, illness and medicine* (pp. 191–204). Palgrave Macmillan.

Flores, G., Abreu, M., Barone, C. P., Bachur, R., & Lin, H. (2012). Errors of medical interpretation and their potential clinical consequences: A comparison of professional versus ad hoc versus no interpreters. *Annals of Emergency Medicine*, *60*(5), 545–553.

Galbally, F. (1978). *Migrant services and programs: Report of the review of postarrival programs and services for migrants.* Australian Government Publishing Service.

Garrett, P. W., Dickson, H. G., Young L., & Klinken Whelan, A. (2008). "The Happy Migrant Effect": Perceptions of negative experiences of healthcare by patients with little or no English: A qualitative study across seven language groups. *Quality Safety Health Care*, *17*, 101–103. https://doi.org/10.1136/qshc.2007.022426

Gilson, M., & Zubrzycki, J. (1967). *The foreign-language press in Australia: 1848–1964.* Australian National University Press.

Grassby, A. J. (1984). *The tyranny of prejudice.* AE Press.

Hage, G. (2002). Multiculturalism and white paranoia in Australia. *Journal of International Migration and Integration/Revue de l'integration et de la migration internationale*, *3*, 417–437.

Hearn, J. M. (1981). *The unrecognised professionals.* Education Research and Development Committee.

Henderson, R. F., Harcourt, A. D., & Harper, R. J. A. (1970). *People in poverty: A Melbourne survey.* Institute of Applied Economic and Social Research.

Hirmiz, I. (2014). Non-accredited interpreters: A lose-lose situation. In *Touch*, *22*(3), 12–13.

Hlavac, J. (2016). Interpreter credentialing, testing and training in Australia: Past, contemporary and future directions. *FITISPos International Journal*, *3*, 59–81. https://doi.org/10.37536/FITISPos-IJ.2016.3.0.98

Hlavac, J. (2021). The development of community translation and interpreting in Australia. In J. Wakabayashi & M. O'Hagan (Eds.), *Translating and interpreting in Australia and New Zealand* (pp. 65–85). Routledge. https://doi.org/10.4324/9781003150770

Hlavac, J., Beagley, J., & Zucchi, E. (2018). Applications of policy and the advancement of patients' health outcomes through interpreting services: Data and viewpoints from a major public healthcare provider. *Translation & Interpreting: The International Journal of Translation and Interpreting Research*, *10*(1), 111–136.

Jordens, A. M. (1993). Communicating with migrants: The development of language teaching and of translating and interpreting services in Australia 1945-75. Working paper no. 12. Research School of Social Sciences, Australian National University, Australia.

Jupp, J. (2002). *From white Australia to Woomera: The story of Australian immigration.* Cambridge University Press.

Jupp, J. (2004). *The English in Australia*. Cambridge University Press.
Kerr, A. (1981). Language and education in a diverse society. In J. Sherwood (Ed.), *Multicultural education: Issues and innovations* (pp. 157–169). Creative Research.
Kerrigan, V., McGrath, S. Y., Majoni, S. W., Walker, M., Ahmat, M., Lee, B., ... & Ralph, A. P. (2021). "The talking bit of medicine, that's the most important bit": Doctors and Aboriginal interpreters collaborate to transform culturally competent hospital care. *International Journal for Equity in Health*, *20*, 1–15. https://doi.org/10.1186/s12939-021-01507-1
Krupinski, J. (1984). Changing patterns of migration to Australia and their influence on the health of migrants. *Social Science & Medicine*, *18*(11), 927–937. https://doi.org/10.1016/0277-9536(84)90263-6
Liddicoat, A. J. (2009). Policy change and educational inertia: Language policy and language education in Australian schooling. In A. J. Liddicoat & A. Scarino (Eds.), *Languages in Australian education: Problems, prospects and future directions* (pp. 11–24). Cambridge Scholars Publishing.
Lo Bianco, J. (1987). *National policy on languages*. Australian Government Publishing Service.
Markus, A., & Taft, M. (2015). Postwar immigration and assimilation: A reconceptualisation. *Australian Historical Studies*, *46*(2), 234–251. https://doi.org/10.1080/1031461X.2015.1035288
Martin, J. I. (1978). *The migrant presence: Australian responses 1947-1977*. Allen & Unwin.
Masterman, G. G., & Wentworth, W. C. (1969). *Poverty in Australia*. Angus and Robertson.
Migrant & Refugee Health Partnership. (2020). *Interpreter Engagement in General Practice in Australia*. https://culturaldiversityhealth.org.au/wp-content/uploads/2020/06/Interpreter-Engagement-in-General-Practice-in-Australia.pdf
Murphy, H. B. M. (1952). The assimilation of refugee immigrants in Australia. *Population Studies*, *5*(3), 179–206.
Ozolins, U. (1985). The national language policy issue in Australia. In M. Clyne (Ed.), *Australia, meeting place of languages* (pp. 281–299). Pacific Linguistics.
Ozolins, U. (1998). *Interpreting and translating in Australia: Current issues and International comparisons*. Language Australia.
Ozolins, U. (2001). Inventiveness and regression: Interpreting/translating and the vicissitudes of Australian language policy. In J. L. Bianco & R. Wickert (Eds.), *Australian policy activism in language and literacy* (pp. 255–278). Language Australia.
Ozolins, U. (2016). T&I practitioners and agencies: Tensions despite a common cause. In *Touch*, *24*(2), 10–11.
Ozolins, U., & Clyne, M. (2001) Immigration and language policy in Australia. In G. Extra & D. Gorter (Eds.), *The other languages of Europe* (pp. 371–90). Multilingual Matters.
Partington, G. (1981). 'Education for a multicultural society': A policy statement and a critique. *Australian Quarterly*, *53*(4), 467–475.

Phillips, C. B., & Travaglia, J. (2011). Low levels of uptake of free interpreters by Australian doctors in private practice: Secondary analysis of national data. *Australian Health Review*, *35*(4), 475–479. https://doi.org/10.1071/AH10900

Pybus, C. (2006). *Black founders: The unknown story of Australia's first black settlers*. UNSW Press.

Rosa, J., & Flores, N. (2017). Unsettling race and language: Toward a raciolinguistic perspective. *Language in Society*, *46*(5), 621–647. https://doi.org/10.1017/S0047404517000562

Saito, S., Harris, M. F., Long, K. M., Lewis, V., Casey, S., Hogg, W., ... & Russell, G. (2021). Response to language barriers with patients from refugee background in general practice in Australia: Findings from the OPTIMISE study. *BMC Health Services Research*, *21*, 1–12. https://doi.org/10.1186/s12913-021-06884-5

Schulz, T. (2020). Successful elements of an improved model of care for refugees and immigrants in regional Australia [Doctoral dissertation, University of Melbourne].

Shoebridge, J. (1980). The unspeakable in pursuit: The Australian health services and its migrants, *Community Health Studies*, *4*(3), 236–241. https://doi.org/10.1111/j.1753-6405.1980.tb00306.x

Showstack, R. (2019). Patients don't have language barriers; The healthcare system does. *Emergency Medicine Journal*, *36*(10), 580–581. https://doi.org/10.1136/emermed-2019-208929

Simpson, J., & Wigglesworth, G. (2019). Language diversity in Indigenous Australia in the 21st century. *Current Issues in Language Planning*, *20*(1), 67–80. https://doi.org/10.1080/14664208.2018.1503389

Smolicz, J. J. (1984). Is the monolingual nation-state out-of-date? A comparative study of language policies in Australia and the Philippines. *Comparative Education*, *20*(2), 265–285. https://doi.org/10.1080/0305006840200207

Translators and Interpreters Australia. (2020). *Many languages – one voice*. https://tia.professionalsaustralia.org.au/Interpreters/What_we_do/Campaigns/Many_language/Interpreters/Campaigns/ML1V.aspx?hkey=9aa4db4f-42f7-401d-9c5f-c6fdd2936167

Vanstone, R., Szwarc, J., Casey, S., Maloney, M., & Duell-Piening, P. (2013). *Promoting the engagement of interpreters in Victorian health services*. Victorian Foundation for Survivors of Torture.

Vickers, A. (1988). Racism and colonialism in early Australian novels about Southeast Asia. *Asian Studies Review*, *12*(1), 7–12. https://doi.org/10.1080/03147538808712533

West, S. (1980, June 15). *New policies, old issues*. Conference on ethnic and immigration studies. NSW. https://parlinfo.aph.gov.au/parlInfo/download/media/pressrel/HNC012017013339/upload_binary/HNC012017013339.pdf;fileType=application%2Fpdf#search=%22media/pressrel/HNC012017013339%22

White, J., Plompen, T., Osadnik, C., Tao, L., Micallef, E., & Haines, T. (2018). The experience of interpreter access and language discordant clinical encounters in Australian health care: A mixed methods exploration. *International Journal for Equity in Health*, *17*, 1–10. https://doi.org/10.1186/s12939-018-0865-2

4 Market monolingualism

4.1 Any bilinguals can interpret

While I was working on this book, I received an email from a person who wanted to set up a private language service provision agency in Australia. Looking for interpreters willing to work for the company, the email explicitly said that "an interpreter's qualification is not necessary". Self-assessed proficiency in English and another language was all that was required. People would not hire someone who might be very good at fixing drains yet does not have a plumber's qualification as a plumber. People would not hire someone who has raised many children yet does not have a relevant qualification as a childcare worker. The same goes for many other jobs. Why then does this basic tenet of professional competence not apply to interpreting?

Becoming a professional interpreter (and a translator) in Australia takes years of hard work. People who wish to become interpreters in Australia need to pass interpreting certification exams administered by NAATI. In order to sit for NAATI-administered exams, candidates must complete an interpreting course at institutions endorsed by NAATI, which takes one to two years depending on the levels of certifications. As the overall pass rate is very low at around 15 per cent (The Migration Translators, 2023), students enrolled in interpreting courses need to work hard, sometimes trying multiple times, to succeed.

Despite the amount of effort and investment it takes to become an interpreter, interpreting experiences problems with professional recognition in Australia. Ambivalent professional status remains a key source of professional dissatisfaction among interpreters in Australia (see Eser & Lai, 2018; Hale & Napier, 2016; Rodriguez-Losada, 2019). A lack of professional recognition of interpreting is, indeed, not limited to Australia. Interpreting requires specialised skills (e.g., cognitive processing, memory retention and note-taking), public speaking abilities and an extensive amount of knowledge across diverse areas. This specialised nature of interpreting is,

DOI: 10.4324/9781032614854-4

however, not well understood by people outside the field, and consequently impacts the professional legitimacy of interpreting (Inghilleri, 2010).

Following a social turn in interpreting (see Section 1.2.1), a growing number of studies have paid attention to the issue of interpreters' status from a sociological perspective (e.g., Cho, 2017; Dam & Zethsen, 2013; Gentile, 2016; Giustini, 2022; Sela-Sheffy, 2010; Tseng, 1992). The literature shows that interpreter status is generally low due to the secondary nature of interpreting work, unsystematic qualification systems, the predominantly freelancing nature of interpreting, a lack of opportunities for career advancement and the concentration of female workers in the field.

While the professional status of interpreters is generally seen as not high, one area grants interpreters, particularly conference interpreters, significant professional recognition in certain societies: language skills. In China, a group of English-Chinese interpreters is positively famous due to the popularity of English language learning (Birtles, 2018). As a global language, English is keenly pursued among Chinese people due to socially recognised forms of material and symbolic benefits from English language competence (Li, 2020). Some interpreters even enjoy celebrity status due to their excellent interpreting and fluent English skills (Cho, 2022). As these interpreters tend to serve high-ranking government officials (e.g., Prime Minister), they frequently receive media spotlight, which adds more glamour to the profession (Du & Wang, 2021).

The ties between the status of a foreign language and the social perception of interpreters are also illustrated in the case of Korean interpreters specialising in English (see Cho, 2017). English language learning there is extremely popular as illustrated by the term *yeongeo yulpung* or 'English fever', due to the instrumental and symbolic value of English in Korean society. As such, interpreters specialising in English are admired for their fluent English and are glamourised as elite bilinguals. Similar to their Chinese counterparts, some English-Korean interpreters have achieved fame on a par with celebrity status (Cho, 2022). Stories regarding the superhuman effort that celebrity interpreters have made to master English are widely circulated in Korean society through various outlets including television, autobiographies, news articles and social media (Cho, 2021). This has, in turn, contributed to the establishment of interpreters as bona fide professionals dedicated to perfection (Cho, 2015).

Similarly, English language learning has been highly popular in Japan, and the language skills of interpreters are well recognised as a distinctive characteristic of interpreting. Foreign language mastery is, indeed, one key motivation behind the pursuit of interpreting particularly among Japanese women keen to exercise autonomy over career building (Bailey, 2006). In particular, conference interpreters specialising in English are socially respected for their fluency in English (Giustini, 2022), illustrating the ties between the socially ascribed value of language and public perception of interpreters.

The high social recognition of interpreters' language skills in those countries comes in sharp contrast to interpreters in Australia who are literally invisible in the society. For one thing, foreign language learning has hardly been valued in the historically English-monolingual Australia (see Chapter 3 for details). Apart from the issue of low societal recognition of language, the type of interpreting also differs between Australia and the countries mentioned above. While community interpreting which helps NESB migrants to manage their daily lives is the mainstream interpreting in Australia, conference interpreting represents the most dominant form of interpreting in those and many other countries. Regarded as the 'stars' of the profession (Dam & Zethsen, 2013), conference interpreters generally enjoy external recognition for their mastery of language and association with the powerful figures they serve (Cho, 2017). Even conference interpreters, however, remain extremely low-profile in Australian society. Interpreting in Australia is an area of sheer public disinterest, with the ambivalent professional status of interpreters remaining as a core occupational issue (Eser & Lai, 2018).

Status is a "context-dependent construct" (Giustini, 2022, p. 6), and it can be presumed that interpreters' status is tied to local sociolinguistic conditions. Building on the historical examination of societal monolingualism in the previous chapter, this chapter investigates how the racial and class-based workings of English monolingualism play out in the interpreting market in contemporary Australia. It approaches interpreters as bilingual migrant workers to examine how societal monolingualism, which disadvantages other languages and speakers, is replicated in the labour market characterised by migrant concentration. In doing so, the chapter emphasises market monolingualism as a key source of inequality for bilingual interpreters, highlighting the need to bring about changes to the monolingual way of seeing bilingualism as a non-skill.

4.2 Migration and interpreting

As illustrated in the previous chapter, interpreting in Australia has long been a profession with a high concentration of migrants working in it. This migrant aspect of interpreting figures prominently in the data under examination too. Out of the 67 participants, only three were Australian-born. The other 64 participants have migrant backgrounds, having arrived in Australia at different times, with 1969 being the earliest year of arrival and 2022 being the latest year to move to Australia.

Table 4.1 shows the demographic details of the participants.

Table 4.1 Participant profiles

Category	*Range*	*Number*	*%*
Place of birth	Australia	3	4.5%
	Elsewhere	64	95.5%
Gender	Male	20	29.9%
	Female	47	70.1%
Education level	PhD	3	4.5%
	Master's	35	52.2%
	Bachelor's	14	20.9%
	Undergraduate	12	17.9%
	Incompletion	2	3.0%
Types of interpreting	Full-Time	35	52.2%
	Part-Time	26	38.8%
	Retirement Job	6	9%

The heavy concentration of migrants in interpreting raises two questions: why has the profession of interpreting continued to be a migrant-concentrated job and how does the migrant aspect of interpreting influence interpreters' engagement with the market? Examining these questions necessitates an understanding of how the participants got into the profession in relation to their migrant status. Analysis of the data extrapolated from the interviews with the participants identifies three primary factors specific to the ties between migration and interpreting.

First, unsuccessful job searching is one factor which led the participants to interpreting. Many migrants in Australia experience challenges finding a job that matches their previous qualifications and skills due to the non-recognition of the overseas qualifications they hold (Tan et al., 2014; Webb, 2015). As migrants are often unable to find a job commensurate with their previous qualifications, those who can speak English well reportedly resort to work that uses their bilingual skills. As a key area which requires bilingual skills, translation and interpreting has served as an interim pathway for migrants in Australia until they find a better alternative (Darwish, 2005). For example, Participant 20, a Swahili interpreter who was an educator in his home country, tried to find a job that matched his previous teaching qualifications upon arriving in Australia. The participant, however, had trouble finding a school teaching position due to the non-recognition of those qualifications and sought interpreting work based on his bilingual skills. It is worth noting that the agency accepted him as an interpreter without requiring any professional qualifications:

> Yeah, when I got here in Australia, it was hard for me to find a job, because they were all asking qualifications, and the qualifications I had at that time were not accepted. But with my languages, I went to the interpreting, translator company. I just explained that I am multilingual, and then I got jobs straightaway, and I started working on a casual basis.
>
> (Participant 20)

Second and relatedly, a sudden demand for interpreting due to the influx of refugees is another key factor which led the participants to the field. As a popular destination for refugees, Australia experiences a constant arrival of refugees most of whom do not speak English. With each wave of refugees, an urgent need arises for interpreters speaking their language. The story of Participant 46, a Tamil interpreter, exemplifies how the unpredictable nature of demand for interpreting influences migrant job seekers to get into interpreting. Similar to the Swahili interpreter mentioned above, the participant looked for a job commensurate with his previous qualifications, to no avail. He was motivated to get into the field when Tamil became a sought-after language after the influx of refugees fleeing from the Sri Lankan Civil War (1983–2009). This participant did not hold any professional interpreting qualification either:

> No, I didn't have [qualifications] actually, so the first six years no, I mean the seventh year, yes. At that time there was a huge demand in interpreting and we had a number of asylum seekers on-site because of the civil war in Sri Lanka.
>
> (Participant 46)

Third, gender was an important element which influenced female migrant participants to pursue interpreting. The gendered dimension of interpreting is demonstrated by the fact that out of the 67 participants, 47 – or more than two-thirds – are female. The feminisation of interpreting is a key characteristic of the profession and is regarded as one reason for its low recognition (Giustini, 2022). The reasons behind the feminisation of interpreting vary, ranging from women's desires for autonomous career building free from gender discrimination (Giustini, 2019) to the flexibility accorded by the freelancing nature of interpreting in terms of balancing work and domestic responsibilities (Cho, 2017). In the case of migrant women, that balance is particularly problematic due to a significant lack of a personal network (e.g., grandparents) important to the management of domestic duties. Many also experience gendered racism in the Anglo-dominant labour market in Australia (Lee, 2005).

The specific circumstances of migrant women are found to push female migrants to seek casual jobs as their only possible career option (see Salaff & Greve, 2003). The case of Participant 42, a Greek interpreter, is a key example:

> For me, what's important at this stage, until my baby starts school, is to be as much as I can be with him. So interpreting is actually ideal, because it's mostly short jobs. Sometimes, it's six, eight hours, but it's not very common. It's not every day, and I have the freedom to say, no, I don't want to take it, my baby's sick today, or yes, I will take it, or whatever.
>
> (Participant 42)

The data analysis illustrates the strong ties between interpreting and migration. It highlights that motivations behind interpreting centre around the distinctive circumstances of migrants characterised by difficulties of finding jobs, influx of migrants and increased domestic responsibilities. Importantly, it characterises interpreting as an area which is isolated from the mainstream, with work predominantly performed by migrants for migrants. With this continued pattern of migrant concentration in interpreting in mind, the next section examines how interpreting is perceived and treated in the local interpreting market in relation to English monolingualism.

4.3 Bilingualism as a non-skill

This section first explores public perceptions of interpreting through the concept of linguistic market (Bourdieu, 1993) to understand how interpreting is socially perceived in contemporary Australia. It then moves on to investigate how interpreting is evaluated in material terms in the language market.

4.3.1 In the linguistic market

Markets have served as key sites of sociolinguistic research and can be both physical and abstract. In the classic sociolinguistic study on department stores conducted by Labov (1972), for example, shops represent a physical domain of "public use of language in everyday life" (p. 49) to understand how different speech communities use language under no explicit observation. Labov's research reveals that the linguistic behaviours of upper-middle-class shoppers were in line with the expectations of the shops that catered to people from higher-class backgrounds. It shows that these shoppers tended to use more standard language forms and exhibited careful speech patterns when interacting with store employees. This behaviour was in line with the shops' expectations, as these establishments often associated standard language use with higher social status. The study illustrates how social stratification dictates speech production, normalising and reinforcing the established class-based language use through everyday practices.

In an abstract sense, the theory of *linguistic market* proposed by Bourdieu (1993) highlights the relations of linguistic hierarchies in which a certain variety of language is more valued than others. In this metaphorical sense of the market, language can be a product that is constantly assessed and judged according to established linguistic relations, with a dominant form of linguistic product securing "*a profit of distinctiveness*" (Bourdieu, 1977, pp. 654, emphasis in original). The linguistic market is inseparable from societal power relations, as power asymmetries result in the distinction between the dominant and dominated languages, and the dominant language is almost invariably the language of the dominant group. Languages and speakers are hierarchised according to the amount of value ascribed to each linguistic product, which, in turn, helps maintain existing power relations (see also Section 2.2).

Applied to Australia, the linguistic market is in favour of English with other languages subordinated to it (see Chapter 3 for details). Data analysis indicates that within this English-centred monolingual milieu, interpreting is found to be generally undervalued. The participants reported that, as a language-focused profession, interpreting is not highly valued due to the low level of prestige attached to language as a professional skill. While it takes a significant amount of investment and hard work to become an interpreter, the amount of work required to master language to be proficient enough to do interpreting is reported to be often not understood by the public who are generally not interested in language learning. This observation is in line with the public disinterest in language learning in Australia. Taking Australian teenagers as an example, Australian students are reported to rank the lowest among OECD countries in terms of their interest in language learning (De Bortoli et al., 2021). The lack of respect for interpreting is well exemplified below:

> Yeah, because yeah, like I said, it's very responsible job and I would like people to respect the interpreters.
>
> (Participant 8, Japanese interpreter)

> There is very little, I would say respect, of interpreters.
>
> (Participant 4, Farsi interpreter)

Similarly, the participants reported that many people see other languages as irrelevant to their lives and this monolingual perspective impacts the ways in which interpreting is perceived as a profession. All too often, interpreting is seen as something that any bilingual can do. Furthermore, the nature of community interpreting in which migrant interpreters serve migrant clients was said to be another key factor which renders interpreting "a very isolated job" in the words of Participant 3, a Farsi interpreter. This lack of understanding about bilingualism and interpreting was reported to be a source of the under-appreciation of interpreting:

> I don't think it [interpreting] is really seen as a profession, like as a profession. It's probably seen as more just really – how to say? It's not seen as a profession. It's just a way of helping the people to communicate with each other. So, and one of the things probably I think in Australia, because they are predominantly, of course, English speaking people, so they don't really take – as you know, average Australian, they will only speak English, not many other languages. So, they don't know, probably they don't appreciate the learning, how hard it is to learn the different language.
>
> (Participant 64, Mongolian interpreter)

The analysis of the interview data indicates that the lack of appreciation for interpreting is not just linguistic but may also be racial and class-based. Research shows that ethnic minorities proficient in the societal language tend to be negatively judged in terms of intelligence and status (Harrison, 2013; Holmes et al., 2001; Kang & Rubin, 2009). No matter how proficient in the dominant language minority individuals are, linguistic minorities are generally stereotyped as less competent than the mainstream due to the entrenched biases against people who look different and speak differently (Holmes et al., 2001). In the case of English, accented speech is strongly associated with minority status, which, in turn, diminishes minority speakers' professional credibility and chances of advancement in the workplace (Harrison, 2013).

These racial and class biases tied to language were reported by many participants. Whilst highly proficient in English, this predominantly migrant group felt they were generally treated as a semi-professional group, if not looked down upon. Importantly, the concentration of migrants in the profession is found to influence its low recognition. The participants reported their impression of interpreting as an isolated profession, which was said to be "seen as not white people's job" and has, therefore, never been valued, according to Participant 67, a Mongolian interpreter. During the interviews, the strong sense of under-recognition was shared by others, as exemplified below:

> Just there's no one respect that this is the field. That people tend to overlook that hey, you know you guys are just an interpreter. You just translate information from one language to another language.
>
> (Participant 29, Bengali interpreter)

At the same time, the analysis of the data indicates that the under-appreciation of interpreting is not always deliberate; it may also be an outcome of unconscious biases relating to English monolingualism. That is, the superiority-inferiority binary between English and other languages and, by extension, English speakers and other language speakers, has been normalised in local consciousness. It is, therefore, only natural for many people to see other languages as unimportant, rather than people actively resisting languages other than English. In this monolingual habitus (Gogolin, 1997), interpreting as a language-based profession does not receive public attention, which, in turn, strengthens its social invisibility. The very nature of interpreting as a job which does not concern the lives of most Australians was also reported as another element which contributes to the normalisation of interpreting as a job for 'the others'. The normalised state of interpreting as an under-recognised profession in English-monolingual Australia is well exemplified by the excerpt below:

> Well, the general – they don't concern themselves with translating and interpreting. Monolingual people don't think about beyond the realm of their own language. They think their language is the only language in the world. They see the need because they are aware other people don't speak English, but we're not highly regarded. I guess we're just like some professional [...] they don't have an understanding or an appreciation. They don't dislike us. They just don't know what it is like.
>
> (Participant 26, Spanish interpreter)

The analysis of the data illustrates that the linguistic relations of dominance established in the linguistic market are responsible for the general under-recognition of the profession of interpreting. In the monolingual social milieu characterised by biases against other language and speakers, language is hardly recognised as a special skill, which, in turn, leads to the general tendency that sees interpreting as a semi-profession. The findings show that as a profession, interpreting continues to be under-appreciated and remains isolated from mainstream life. With this in mind, the next section examines how the profession of interpreting is valuated in the material terms in the Australian interpreting market.

4.3.2 In the language market

Following the rise of linguistic commodification in recent years, sociolinguists have argued for the need to reapproach the idea of 'market' (see McGill, 2013). The theory of linguistic commodification posits that language has become commodified as a product linked to the economic and cultural processes in the context of the globalised new economy (Heller et al., 2014). According to this theory, languages that are sought-after (e.g., English, Chinese, etc.) have become commodities which have high transactional value in the global market (Holborow, 2018). Workers proficient in those languages have distinctive advantages in the sale and service areas, for example, which demonstrates the reconfiguration of language as an economic resource (Holborow, 2018). While acknowledging the usefulness of linguistic commodification in the framing of language as an economic resource, some scholars have argued for the need to pay attention to the monetary value of language traded in the market (Kelly-Holmes, 2016): if language has indeed become a commodity, it should then be possible to examine its actual monetary exchange.

The call for attention to the monetary value of language is particularly relevant to interpreting in which bilingual proficiency represents a core skill of the profession. Unlike other professions in which language constitutes a subset of job qualifications (e.g., a salesperson capable of speaking another language), interpreting requires language as the most important professional skill. Unlike many other professions which require language skills, interpreting in Australia has a high concentration of migrants. Examination of the financial remuneration for migrant-background interpreters in the Australian interpreting market is, therefore, expected to reveal the potentially racialised and class-based workings of the language market.

To begin with, data analysis indicates a general sense of interpreting as an underpaid job and a strong sense of professional under-valuation felt by the participants. Nearly all participants expressed dissatisfaction with the market rates for interpreting, with many reporting that it is almost unsustainable to make a living out of the profession. While the five interpreters working full-time for public hospitals appeared to be generally happy with job security and regularity of income, the view of interpreting as an underpaid profession was also shared by those participants. Money as a source of demotivation is illustrated by the following interview excerpts by Participant 39, who works as a full-time interpreter for a hospital:

> I think it's shameful what we get paid for the job we do, I really do. I mean we have such a huge responsibility. I mean we are talking about the health of people, mental health, physical health. We have a huge

> responsibility and we are paid as, you know, anybody who doesn't have a professional degree or certificate. We are just absolutely not paid enough and not considered the way we should be and that really hurts.
>
> (Participant 39, Italian interpreter)

The idea of interpreting as an underpaid profession was shared strongly by the participants who worked as freelance interpreters too. To understand how payment for freelance interpreting works in detail, readers need to know there are broadly two types of interpreting services: on-site interpreting in which interpreters travel to provide face-to-face interpreting and remote interpreting enabled by technology such as telephone and video interpreting. At the time of the interviews, all participants were engaged in both modes of interpreting.

Table 4.2 provides an overview of the current market rate for on-site and telephone interpreting based on the data from the interviews in 2022.

At a first glance, the rate appears to be much higher than the national minimum hourly rate of $23.23 (Fair Work Ombudsman, 2024). Data analysis, however, indicates several factors which impact the monetary aspects of interpreting. First, work opportunities are constrained by the freelancing nature of interpreting and demand for language. As illustrated in Table 4.1, around half of the 67 participants (52.2 per cent) reported interpreting as their full-time job, yet only five of them had full-time interpreter positions at government-run public hospitals; the rest of the participants were freelancing on a full-time basis. While full-time interpreter positions at health care institutions provide job security and employee benefits (e.g., paid

Table 4.2 Interpreting rate in Australian market

Interpreting mode	*Standard interpreting rate*		*Extra rate*
On-site interpreting	60 minutes $40–$62	90 minutes $70-$90	$25–$40 for second hour or $10 per 15 minutes
Telephone interpreting	15 minutes $7–$17	60 minutes $25–$40	$7–$10 per 15 minutes or ¢50–$1 per minute

leave), such opportunities are found to be available only for interpreters serving large migrant communities due to the high demand for languages. Conversely, interpreters serving small migrant communities are denied opportunities to secure this more prestigious form of employment due to the low demand for interpreting. As Participant 35, an Arabic interpreter who was based in South Australia at the time of the interview, reported, "there's no need for having an interpreter sit for hours when they might see one or two clients" due to the relatively smaller migrant population in South Australia, compared with other states.

Second, demand for interpreting has declined over the years. Many participants from European backgrounds described their languages as 'dying languages' in the Australian community context, with their main clientele – elderly people with little English – having shrunk over the years. According to Participant 57, a Polish interpreter, for example, he has only one job during the day in two-thirds of the year. He commented during the interview: "It is very difficult for an interpreter to make a living out of that particular profession". Similar observations were made by interpreters specialising in languages such as Mongolian and Tibetan, in which demand for language services is not constant.

Third, competition for interpreting jobs, particularly languages that are in high demand, was high. The participants specialising in high-demand languages (e.g., Mandarin, Thai, Vietnamese, etc.) reported that the market is saturated and interpreters compete for jobs that have declined in recent years. Taking interpreter positions in immigration detention centres as an example, the participants said that these positions are often full-time (for a fixed term) and pay well and the relatively good working conditions have attracted many interpreters to detention centres. With the Australian borders tightening for refugees in recent years, however, such jobs are said to have declined significantly. Compounded by the period of Australian border closure during the COVID-19 pandemic, the drop in the intake of migrants and refugees has had similar impact on many participants, who "have to be on call 24/7" (Participant 26, Spanish interpreter), in a system where getting work relies on being the first available interpreter.

Fourth, working conditions for interpreters were said to have deteriorated over the years. The lack of continuity and resultant financial impact are found to be compounded by the expectations that interpreters should be responsible for work-related expenses. As can be seen in Table 4.2, on-site interpreting pays better than remote interpreting. Many participants, however, expressed their hesitation to take up on-site interpreting work due to the general non-coverage of work-related expenses such as travel time and parking fees. This, in turn, pushes interpreters to resort to remote interpreting jobs, despite the lower pay rate for them. The struggles of interpreters are well exemplified by the following narrative:

> That is not cool at all. We're the one who are at the frontline and providing them with information. Please consider the travel costs, the costs of carparking. There's no free hospital carpark. We need to pay for our own carpark. The cost of petrol. You know nowadays petrol, is increasing. It's expensive. Everything is increasing. Food, groceries. You go to Woolworths and Coles. Everything is up but our payment is not up at all. It's still the same. We're still the same for like what? I've been working professionally for three years. This three years is the same. There's no increasing fee or anything.
>
> (Participant 56, Cambodian interpreter)

The market principle of expenses as the interpreter's responsibility is found to be justified by the increasing market treatment of interpreters as independent contractors, rather than employees. Following the government restructuring of interpreting in the late-20th century, work-related expenses which had previously been covered by employers became interpreter responsibilities (see Section 3.4). With the dismantling of full-time interpreter positions in government agencies, many interpreters freelance as subcontractors who are expected to be self-responsible for work-related expenses. According to Participant 26, an Arabic interpreter with over 25 years of interpreting experience, working conditions have continued to deteriorate over past decades:

> Since I started, say 1990, something like that, they used to pay us petrol. They used to pay us for time, travel time, plus the job. We used to earn good money, so I would go anywhere. Go from my home to the east to the west, it didn't affect me. Now, we are getting less and we are not paid for travel time or petrol.
>
> (Participant 26)

While the interpreting rate is already low, it has hardly increased over many years, with rates having rather declined in some cases. According to Participant 7, a Farsi interpreter, the interpreter has received the same rate of nine dollars for 15-minute telephone interpreting work for 12 years, and this story resonated with many other participants. Some participants reported that they are now paid by the minute for telephone interpreting, rather than a flat fee for the standard allocated time of 15 minutes. A deterioration in the working conditions is aptly illustrated by the experience of Participant 40, a Dari-Hazaragi interpreter:

Interpreter: They [an agency] did send a new agreement and I [blindly] signed it and I send it but I didn't know what they'd done. I looked in my case list. I interpreted for a person for five minutes and they paid me $4.
Researcher: Oh, they went by minute?
Interpreter: Yeah. They paid me $4. Then the other one, there was two minutes. They paid me $1.50. I got very disappointed with this.

The economic consequences faced by interpreters contrast with the educational qualifications of the participants. When interpreting was formalised in the 1970s, no tertiary education course specialised in interpreting in Australia. As such, training and education were not a requirement for interpreter qualifications. With the incorporation of interpreting (and translation) studies into Australian tertiary education, however, the level of education held by interpreters has improved over time. This is demonstrated by the education received by the participants. At the time of the interviews, only two participants did not have tertiary education, with 26 participants holding undergraduate or bachelor's degrees, 35 having master's degrees and three having PhD degrees (see Table 4.1). While better education is anticipated to be rewarded with higher financial returns, it seems to be hardly the case with the participants.

Analysis of the data reveals that the market practices are not just economic but social, revealing that the low monetary value attached to interpreting is attributable to English monolingualism and the concentration of migrants in interpreting. Market monolingualism, which devalues language as a skill, is well exemplified by the practice of hiring any bilingual person as an interpreter. It was reported that the idea of 'any bilinguals can interpret', which is widely believed in Australian society, is widespread in the interpreting market too. All too often, interpreters' qualifications are not required for employment (see also Section 4.2). During the interviews, frustration over the market practice of using unqualified bilinguals as interpreters was commonly expressed by the participants. For example:

> The agency doesn't care whether the interpreter is accredited or not. The agency got the commission on the jobs we did, the interpreter did. If I can't take the job, they can get someone to take the job. He's got the same pay with me. Even though I got accreditation, it's not really much incentive.
>
> (Participant 43, Burmese interpreter)

The analysis of narratives indicates that the monolingual bias of bilingualism as a non-skill and the low financial treatment of interpreting have been sustained by the racial and class dimensions of interpreting as a migrant-concentrated profession. As examined in Section 4.2, migrants generally experience problems finding jobs in the process of settlement. Bilingual migrants desperate for money are attracted to interpreting and the ease of entering the market has ensured a constant supply of 'interpreters' over the years. The vulnerability of migrant job seekers is exploited by the market, which, in turn, sustains ongoing devaluation of interpreting. The market practice of taking advantage of migrants was bemoaned by many participants during the interviews:

> Now if somebody doesn't have any other qualification and a normal cleaner or say service station attendant, they may be willing to work for $30 an hour or $40 an hour. So, they [agencies] don't distinguish between whether they are doing cleaning or whether they are doing interpreting.
>
> (Participant 34, Hindi interpreter)

It is worth noting how market monolingualism affects not just interpreters but vulnerable groups that interpreters serve. The participants reported that in some urgent cases, unqualified bilinguals whose language did not match that of the other party were hired as 'interpreters' just for the sake of interpreting. The experience of Participant 11, a Rohingya interpreter, is a case in point. When asked how he got into interpreting, the participant said that he was looking for a job and found an interpreter recruitment advertisement by an interpreting agency which was recruiting interpreters to be sent to an overseas refugee detention centre. Anyone who was interested in the job was reported to be hired, with no requirement for either qualifications or proof of bilingual proficiency. When he arrived at the centre, the participant reported witnessing people interpreting in a language in which they lacked proficiency. Examples include a person from a Rohingya background interpreting for an Arabic-speaking refugee and an Afghan-background person interpreting for a Farsi-speaking refugee. This was despite the potentially huge consequences of misinterpreting on the fate of refugees who had risked their lives for the slim chances of starting a new life in the new country. The example of Participant 11, once again, highlights the market practice of using any bilinguals for interpreting and the exploitation of migrants in desperate situations.

While the need for the reform of the language market was emphasised by the participants, the minority status of interpreters and the profession is found to be a significant obstacle to such reforms. As a profession which consists of many different ethnic groups and freelancing practitioners, interpreting was reported as lacking sufficient force to form significant bargaining power to change the market practices. The limited amount of power accorded to interpreters as minority groups is well illustrated by the following excerpt:

> The state government's [does not] really look upon interpreters as a significant population, even if they go on and there's more collectivity. There is this couple of major unions. The bargaining power is not very big enough for them to force the hand of the government. It's a significant minority. So, from time to time there have been bits and pieces given, but I haven't seen in the last 12 years any big upswing in the way I've been paid.
>
> (Participant 46, Tamil interpreter)

Data analysis indicates interpreting as a space of double minority. On the one hand, interpreters are mostly migrants coming from minority backgrounds. On the other hand, the profession is inherently disparate because it is composed of workers who come from widely different cultural backgrounds and predominantly freelance. This minority aspect of interpreting is conjectured to be one reason behind the continued poor treatment of interpreters by the market.

Analysis of the data also illustrates that market monolingualism is sustained and strengthened by the racial and class-based dimension of interpreting as a migrant-concentrated profession. Untrained bilinguals working as interpreters in the Australian interpreting market are often blamed for disrupting the state of the market (see Rodriguez-Losada, 2019). The findings, however, show that it is not individuals who should be blamed but the exploitative market that needs to be held responsible for ongoing under-recognition of interpreting.

4.4 Reconciling with reality

Following the examination of the market treatment of interpreters, this section explores how individual interpreters respond to the market's practices. Our conversations identify the poor recognition of interpreting as a primary source of professional disempowerment. The participants reported feelings of devaluation and even helplessness at the ways in which interpreters are treated in professional terms. For example:

> But as I say, the organisation doesn't care about all this educational background, and I'm equivalent to the person who hasn't done any of these things and doesn't have any debt for her loan or from her studies. I'm a big loser. I'm no different to that person to the government. I'm nobody. I'm doing my job better than anybody else. Who cares?
>
> (Participant 3, Farsi interpreter)

While some participants reported a plan to transition to another career due to the lack of interpreting work and unsustainably low market rate, data analysis indicates that many participants were generally trying to reconcile with the market by managing the issue in a way that suits them best. Analysis identifies three ways to reconcile with market practices: interpreting as a part-time job; gendered compromise; and interpreting as a retirement job.

First, the participants reported that they keep interpreting part-time, while having a full-time job to secure a stable source of income. At the time of the interviews, 26 participants or 38.8 per cent of the cohort had a full-time job (see Table 4.1). While these participants expressed love for interpreting as a dynamic activity and a way of helping others (see Section 6.2), doing interpreting full-time was said to be financially unsustainable. It was particularly so, considering the general struggle of settlement and the Australian labour market which tends to discriminate migrant workers (see Kosny et al., 2017). Many participants, therefore, made the decision to balance financial needs and personal interest by keeping interpreting as a part-time job. The words of Participant 47, a part-time Urdu interpreter, "I have a family, I have a house, I have a mortgage, I have bills, I have a dog, I have cat, I have a car, I have friends, I socialise with friends as well", indicate the improbability of maintaining his lifestyle with income from interpreting alone.

Second, data analysis identifies gender as a key factor behind the participants' acceptance of the status quo as a migrant woman. As illustrated in Section 4.2, migrant women tend to bear more domestic responsibilities due to the lack of personal networks. For those participants who wish to balance work and family, the freelancing nature of interpreting accords them the flexibility which is essential to manage careers while fulfilling carer responsibilities. For this group of participants, interpreting represents a rare opportunity to pursue balanced female lives. The gendered nature of the compromise on market practices is exemplified by the following narrative:

> So, it makes it easy, it makes it easy and, yeah, it's a good job. It earns me a bit of extra income and I usually choose my hours, which I like. I don't have to work a full day if I don't want to. If I have something on, I can block and I cannot accept a job and there's no issue at all.
>
> (Participant 35, Arabic interpreter)

Finally, interpreting was reported as a retirement job by a group of participants who had retired from their full-time job. At the time of the interviews, a total of six participants were engaged in interpreting as a retirement job (see Table 4.1). Five of them had previously been engaged in professions unrelated to interpreting yet returned to the field after retirement for the specific purpose of helping vulnerable members of the community (see also Section 6.2). Taking Participant 19, a Japanese interpreter, as an example, the interpreter had previously worked in a high-paying corporate position yet decided to pursue interpreting when she retired. When asked why she wanted to go back to interpreting, she specifically mentioned the desire to help others. For this group of participants, money was reportedly not a primary concern, and the participants tried to distance themselves from other active interpreters. For example:

> They [interpreters] do feel perhaps belittled or ignored but I don't. I just translate and, again, I don't do it as a living. I'm not dependent upon it in any way. I do it as a service.
>
> (Participant 58, Hebrew interpreter)

The deployment of one's language and expertise as a moral obligation which has nothing to do with the material conditions of working as interpreters may have the counter-intuitive effect of sustaining the structural inequalities of the interpreting market. While it is not the intention of this chapter to problematise the effort made by individual interpreters, it is worth considering how the individual-level effort unaccompanied by macro-level responses may sustain and perpetuate structural problems embedded in the interpreting market. From the perspective of the market, those interpreters who value interpreting as a rewarding experience may represent a reliable source of labour unaffected by the material conditions. As long as demand for interpreting is filled by good-willed individuals, the market may find little motivation to change the current practice.

Data analysis illustrates that the participants try to reconcile with the market practices in relation to their migrant circumstances and individually held values. Migration and the migrant status of interpreters figure prominently as a significant factor behind their attempts at reconciliation. First, the financial struggles of many migrants in Australia are found to lead many participants to pursue interpreting part-time. Second, interpreting represents a gendered compromise in the case of female participants whose migrant status makes it difficult to establish a full career in the local labour market. Third, interpreting represents an ideal retirement job for community-minded bilinguals willing to help out NESB migrants.

Similar to the ways in which the participants got into the field (see Section 4.2), the distinctive circumstances of migrants and related social views are found to influence the participants in trying to reconcile with the market realities. The willingness to accommodate the market conditions may, however, work to strengthen and reinforce the very market practices which devalue interpreting. The strong ties between migration and interpreting represent both the cause and effect of the under-valuation of interpreting in the market, which is deeply entrenched in monolingual biases against other languages and speakers.

4.5 Summary

The chapter has examined the racial and class-based dimensions of market monolingualism which impact health care interpreters in Australia. By paying attention to the concentration of migrants in interpreting, it shows how and why interpreting and interpreters are undervalued in the market, which is embedded in English monolingualism tied to linguistic, racial and class biases. The close relationship between migration and interpreting both causes and results from the market's under-valuation of interpreting, which is rooted in monolingual prejudices against other languages and their speakers. The chapter has made three significant findings.

First, the chapter highlights the isolated nature of community interpreting which remains socially invisible and is generally seen as irrelevant to mainstream life. Analysis indicates that the key to that isolation is the concentration of migrants in interpreting in which the work is predominantly performed by migrants for migrants. The social invisibility of interpreting is also reinforced by the traditionally monolingual environment of Australia in which other languages receive hardly any public attention. This contrasts those societies in which interpreters are socially respected due to their bilingual skills, particularly in English (see Section 4.1). The findings highlight strong ties between migration, social invisibility of interpreting and monolingualism, and demonstrate how societal monolingualism is a significant factor in the under-appreciation of interpreting.

Second, the findings illuminate strong ties between societal monolingualism and market monolingualism. From the perspective of the linguistic market, the linguistic relations of dominance established in the unified market have worked to devalue other languages, which, in turn, has negatively influenced social perceptions of interpreting. Macro-societal ideologies are found to influence market practices too, as exemplified by the dominant view that 'any bilinguals can do interpreting'. This belief is not new; it began right from the start of the interpreting profession in English-monolingual Australia (see Chapter 3). The identified market practice of using any bilinguals for interpreting and the resultant devaluation of interpreting are found to strongly relate to societal monolingualism, which has been pervasive in Australia.

Third, the chapter demonstrates how the migrant concentration in interpreting provides fertile ground for market monolingualism to thrive. As amply demonstrated, interpreters are poorly treated by the market, which sees bilingualism as a non-skill. The poor treatment of interpreters is reinforced by the vulnerability of migrants who often have problems finding a job commensurate with their previous qualifications. The ease of entering the market in which professional qualifications are often not required is also found to encourage bilingual migrants to satisfy the demand. While the market is seen to exploit the migrant workers, the disparate nature of the profession of interpreting in which workers come from different ethnic backgrounds and generally freelance is found to make it hard to bring about collective power for change. For these reasons, the vicious cycle of the interpreting market continues, and the findings highlight the urgent need to bring about changes to ongoing market practices.

Considering the identified ties between societal ideologies and market practices, it is important to summon macro-level responses to promote public education on linguistic diversity and the important roles that interpreters play to enhance social equity and equality. Promoting social equity for marginalised populations necessitates cooperation from mainstream society, and awareness is the first step to advancing justice for minority groups including interpreters in multicultural Australia.

References

Bailey, K. (2006). Marketing the eikaiwa wonderland: Ideology, akogare, and gender alterity in English conversation school advertising in Japan. *Environment and Planning D: Society and Space*, *24*(1), 105–130. https://doi.org/10.1068/d418

Birtles, B. (2018, May 31). *Are Interpreters the Key to a Smooth Relationship with China?*. www.abc.net.au/radio/programs/am/are-interpreters-the-key-to-a-smooth-relationship-with-china/10674688

Bourdieu, P. (1977). The economics of linguistic exchanges. *Social Science Information*, *16*(6), 645–668. http://doi:10.1177/053901847701600601

Bourdieu, P. (1993). *Sociology in question*. Sage.

Cho, J. (2015). Sleepless in Seoul: Neoliberalism, English fever, and linguistic insecurity among Korean interpreters. *Multilingua*, *34*(5), 687–710. https://doi.org/10.1515/multi-2013-0047

Cho, J. (2017). *English language ideologies in Korea: Interpreting the past and present*. Springer.

Cho, J. (2021). Neoliberalism and the global spread of English: A Korean case. In B. Schneider, & T. Heyd (Eds.), *Bloomsbury world Englishes* (pp. 142–155). Bloomsbury Publishing. https://doi.org/10.5040/9781350065833.0016

Cho, J. (2022). Hidden gems: Translators and interpreters in Australia play a critical if seldom seen role. *The Conversation*. https://theconversation.com/hidden-gems-translators-and-interpreters-in-australia-play-a-critical-if-seldom-seen-role-188603

Dam, H. V., & Zethsen, K. K. (2013). Conference interpreters—The stars of the translation profession? A study of the occupational status of Danish EU interpreters as compared to Danish EU translators. *Interpreting*, *15*(2), 229–259. https://doi.org/10.1075/intp.15.2.04dam

Darwish, A. (2005). The translation profession in Australia: Viability or survivability?. *Translation Watch Quarterly*, *1*, 82–92.

De Bortoli, L., Underwood, C., & Richardson, S. (2021). *Australian 15-year-old students living in an integrated world.* Australian Council for Educational Research. https://research.acer.edu.au/ozpisa/53

Du, Y., & Wang, B. (2021). A multi-dimensional analysis of the representation of conference interpreters in Chinese media. *Translation Spaces*, *10*(2), 306–328. https://doi.org/10.1075/ts.18011.du

Eser, O., & Lai, M. (2018). Interview with Niki Baras, translators and interpreters Australia–A division of Professionals Australia. *International Journal of Interpreter Education*, *10*(2), 73–78.

Fair Work Ombudsman. (2024). *Minimum Wages.* www.fairwork.gov.au/tools-and-resources/fact-sheets/minimum-workplace-entitlements/minimum-wages

Gentile, P. (2016). *The interpreter's professional status. A sociological investigation into the interpreting profession* [Doctoral dissertation, Università degli Studi di Trieste].

Giustini, D. (2019). 'I thought I could get away from gender discrimination': Linguistic instrumentalism and self-actualisation of female interpreters in temporary employment in Japan. *Japan Forum*, *33*(4), 522–552. https://doi.org/10.1080/09555803.2019.1687566

Giustini, D. (2022). Haken conference interpreters in Japan: Exploring status through the sociology of work and of professions. *Interpreting and Society*, *2*(1), 3–31. https://doi.org/10.1177/27523810211057447

Gogolin, I. (1997). The "monolingual habitus" as the common feature in teaching in the language of the majority in different countries. *Per Linguam: A Journal of Language Learning*, *13*(2), 38–49. https://doi.org/10.5785/13-2-187

Hale, S. B., & Napier, J. (2016). "We're just kind of there": Working conditions and perceptions of appreciation and status in court interpreting. *Target*, *28*(3), 351–371. https://doi.org/10.1075/target.28.3.01hal

Harrison, G. (2013). "Oh, you've got such a strong accent": Language identity intersecting with professional identity in the human services in Australia. *International Migration*, *51*(5), 192–204. https://doi.org/10.1111/imig.12005

Heller, M., Pujolar, J., & Duchêne, A. (2014). Linguistic commodification in tourism. *Journal of Sociolinguistics*, *18*(4), 539–566. https://doi.org/10.1111/josl.12082

Holborow, M. (2018). Language, commodification and labour: The relevance of Marx. *Language Sciences*, *70*, 58–67. https://doi.org/10.1016/j.langsci.2018.02.002

Holmes, K., Murachver, T., & Bayard, D. (2001). Accent, appearance, and ethnic stereotypes in New Zealand. *New Zealand Journal of Psychology*, *30*(2), 79–86.

Inghilleri, M. (2010). "You don't make war without knowing why." The decision to interpret in Iraq. *The Translator*, *16*(2), 175–196. https://doi.org/10.1080/13556509.2010.10799468

Kang, O., & Rubin, D. L. (2009). Reverse linguistic stereotyping: Measuring the effect of listener expectations on speech evaluation. *Journal of Language and Social Psychology*, *28*(4), 441–456. https://doi.org/10.1177/0261927X09341950

Kelly-Holmes, H. (2016). Theorizing the market in sociolinguistics. In N. Coupland (Ed.), *Sociolinguistics: Theoretical debates* (pp. 157–172). Cambridge University Press.

Kosny, A., Santos, I., & Reid, A. (2017). Employment in a "land of opportunity?" Immigrants' experiences of racism and discrimination in the Australian workplace. *Journal of International Migration and Integration*, *18*(2), 483–497. https://doi.org/10.1007/s12134-016-0482-0

Labov, W. (1972). *Sociolinguistic patterns*. University of Pennsylvania Press.

Lee, J. G.-S. (2005). *A narrative analysis of the labour market experiences of Korean migrant women in Australia* [Doctoral dissertation, The University of Sydney].

Li, H. (2020). Changing status, entrenched inequality: How English language becomes a Chinese form of cultural capital. *Educational Philosophy and Theory*, *52*(12), 1302–1313. https://doi.org/10.1080/00131857.2020.1738922

McGill, K. (2013). Political economy and language: A review of some recent literature. *Journal of Linguistic Anthropology*, *23*(2), 196–213.

Rodriguez-Losada, D. (2019). Working conditions as a translator/interpreter in Australia: A personal overview. In A. Armando, I. Öztürk, & D. Aliu (Eds.), *Conceiving migration and communication in a global perspective* (pp. 21–29). Cambridge Scholars Publishing.

Salaff, J., & Greve. A. (2003). Gendered structural barriers to job attainment for skilled Chinese emigrants in Canada. *International Journal of Population Geography*, *9*(6), 443–456. https://doi.org/10.1002/ijpg.310

Sela-Sheffy, R. (2010). "Stars" or "professionals": The imagined vocation and exclusive knowledge of translators in Israel. *MonTI. Monografías de Traducción e Interpretación*, *2*, 131–152. https://doi.org/10.6035/MonTI.2010.2.7

Tan, Y., Rudd, D., & Lester, L. (2024). Employment, income, and skill alignment of humanitarian migrants in the Australian labour market: Metropolitan and regional contexts, 2000–2016. *Geographical Research*, *62*(1), 76–96. https://doi.org/10.1111/1745-5871.12621

The Migration Translators. (2023, December 30). *Why Is It So Easy to Fail the NAATI Translation and Interpreting Tests?*. www.migrationtranslators.com.au/why-is-it-so-easy-to-fail-the-naati-translation-and-interpreting-tests/#:~:text=The%20overall%20average%20pass%20rate,the%20required%20level%20of%20achievement

Tseng, J. (1992). Interpreting as an emerging profession in Taiwan: A sociological model [Master's dissertation, Fu Jen Catholic University].

Webb, S. (2015). 'It's who you know not what': Migrants' encounters with regimes of skills as misrecognition. *Studies in Continuing Education*, *37*(3), 267–285. https://doi.org/10.1080/0158037X.2015.1007938

5 Institutional monolingualism

5.1 Underuse of free interpreting provision

Language barriers pose significant challenges to people unable to speak the dominant language of the host society and are particularly problematic in areas which have life-threatening implications such as health care. Australia is regarded as a global leader in terms of national approaches to language barriers in health care thanks to its nationwide free telephone interpreting service (Bischoff, 2020). Various innovations have been achieved, including the Medical Practitioner Priority Line, which runs 24 hours a day, seven days a week. Interpreting requests on the platform are given priority, and an interpreter will generally be available within three minutes for common languages (Department of Social Services, n.d.a). This free interpreting service is, however, significantly underused in Australian hospitals, and failure to involve an interpreter for NESB patients sometimes results in grave consequences.

Bird (2010) illustrates the serious impact of the non-engagement of interpreters with a story about a 35-year-old Afghan woman. The patient who spoke very little English visited a clinic due to pains in her left leg, accompanied by her 15-year-old daughter as an interpreter. The daughter was, however, only slightly more proficient in English than her mother. On examination, the general practitioner (GP) thought that the patient may have deep vein thrombosis (DVT), which occurs when a clot travels to the lung. The doctor told the daughter that there might be a serious clot in her mother's leg and that she needed to go immediately to a local hospital or a radiology clinic to see if a clot was affecting her leg. The GP wrote a referral for an ultrasound examination and a letter that the patient could take to the hospital, believing that the daughter had understood his advice and instructions. Unfortunately, however, the daughter did not.

Two days following the consultation, the patient died from an extensive DVT while waiting for other family members who were more proficient in English to explain the information provided by the GP. The family believed

DOI: 10.4324/9781032614854-5

that engaging an interpreter would have ensured proper understanding and treatment of the condition and lodged a complaint against the GP. In his response letter to the Medical Board, the GP said that he was unaware of the interpreting service, and he believed that the daughter had understood the instructions during the consultation. The letter further stated that the GP had familiarised himself with the interpreting service since receiving the complaint and that he was now aware of the benefits of engaging a professional interpreter. The Medical Board subsequently closed the matter.

This incident is a clear reflection of two significant problems which have long impacted the use of interpreting in Australian health care. First, interpreting as an essential tool to facilitate communication with NESB patients has long been under-recognised in Australian hospitals (see Sections 3.3 and 3.4). Free interpreting services are available, yet according to the report *Interpreter Engagement in General Practice in Australia* (Migrant & Refugee Health Partnership, 2020), the free interpreting services are used in as little as 1 per cent of consultations with NESB patients. In another study on interpreting service provision for NESB patients during hospital admissions (Blay et al., 2018), interpreters were required in 15.7 per cent of admissions, yet only 3.7 per cent of patients could access interpreter services. Studies on the underuse of health care interpreters in Australia generally view the low uptake of interpreting as systemic issues such as booking complexities and budgets (see Section 3.4). The clinical approaches to the under-utilisation of interpreting, however, overlook the fundamental problems relating to provider awareness of interpreting and the importance of communication with patients from minority backgrounds.

In a study on Australian GP perceptions of interpreting (Bayram et al., 2016), for example, GPs who did not involve interpreters in consultations with NESB patients were asked if using interpreters would have helped improve the quality of the consultations. Only 8.6 per cent of the respondents said that interpreter-aided consultations would have improved in quality; in as many as 89 per cent of consultations, respondents reported that involving an interpreter would have been unlikely to improve quality of care or would have been inappropriate. Indeed, the need for health care interpreting is often not acknowledged in Australian hospitals (Garrette, 2008) and requests for interpreting are seen as burdensome by many hospitals in Australia (Au et al., 2021).

Relatedly and secondly, the case of the Afghan woman exposes the long-standing bias in Australian health care that any bilingual can interpret. Distinctions between professional interpreters and people who are bilingual have always been blurred in Australian hospitals (see Section 3.4). Migrants capable of managing day-to-day conversation are not necessarily familiar with domain-specific terminologies and would, therefore, have trouble understanding complex medical information (Cheng et al., 2021). This aspect of bilingualism is, however, generally not understood by health care staff as exemplified by the common use of bilingual family members or friends as interpreters in Australia (Bayram et al., 2016). This is despite adverse outcomes caused by communication failures such as misunderstanding of diagnoses, increased stress on patients, high hospitalisation and readmission rates (Migrant & Refugee Health Partnership, 2020) and deaths of patients as discussed above.

While the use of lay people as interpreters is not specific to Australia and is widespread in other countries too, it is important to note that Australia is the only country in the Anglophone world which provides a free interpreting service for people not proficient in the dominant language (Phillips & Travaglia, 2011). Understanding the identified pattern of not using the freely available service, which is critical for access equity, necessitates a deeper examination of underlying problems relating to institutional awareness of interpreting and communication with NESB patients.

This chapter, therefore, examines how interpreters are perceived and treated within the traditionally monolingual context of Australian hospitals. In order to capture the holistic picture of institutional perception and treatment of interpreting, it concentrates on front desk staff, doctors and hospital systems.

5.2 Front desk staff as gatekeepers

Patients not proficient in the dominant language often encounter gatekeepers in the process of accessing care. In health care, a number of people are in the position of controlling access to resources, knowledge and services and they include doctors, nurses, front desk staff and policymakers (Collyer et al., 2017). While front desk staff are identified as gatekeepers, there is a significant lack of research on the gatekeeping roles they play in relation to interpreter service arrangement. This section examines common challenges encountered by health care interpreters in their interactions with front desk staff.

In Australia, various states and territories adopt guidelines on working with interpreters, which emphasise the importance of assessing a patient's English language skills carefully. Taking the NSW Health Care Interpreter Service as an example, its assessment process cautions against making hasty assumptions about a patient's English language proficiency based on simple conversations (e.g., about the weather) because the often-complex nature of clinical communication requires far greater proficiency (Health Care Interpreter Service, n.d.).

The ABC Tool developed by the Health Care Interpreter Service identifies three important steps in arranging for an interpreter. As for the first step, 'Assess', hospitals are recommended to determine whether the patient can fully understand and communicate in a medical situation by asking questions relating to current and past medical conditions. Once a need for an interpreter is determined, the next step, 'Booking', identifies the patient's language, a type of interpreting service (e.g., face-to-face, telephone or video) and preferred gender of interpreter. The final stage of 'Confirm' requires recording all booking details in the patient's file and relevant electronic documentation. While the protocol does not specify who should be responsible for language assessment and interpreter arrangement, reception staff members who are the face of hospitals are often the people expected to assess a patient's English language proficiency (Quick, 2024). Their understanding of communication and interpreting is, therefore, pivotal in ensuring proper engagement of interpreters for NESB patients.

Our conversations with interpreters reveal the perception of interpreting among front desk staff as problematic. Rather than following the protocols for interpreter engagement, it was reported that many receptionists look for readily available help for communication management such as asking a bilingual family member or a friend to interpret. This is exemplified by a narrative from Participant 10, a Spanish interpreter:

> Interpreter: You still have admin people saying, bring a friend with you. Bring a member that can help you with the language. You still have that.
>
> Researcher: Even now?
>
> Interpreter: Even now. Even though that there is policy in the health department that says, no you have to use an interpreter. But you still have the admin staff, the receptionist, saying bring someone that will help you.

As reported by this and many other participants, using family members or friends as an interpreter represents a significant health risk, because apparently fluent speakers of English are often unable to understand complex medical communication. The risk of asking lay people to interpret is clearly identified and acknowledged in official guidelines on working with interpreters too. Taking the guidelines published by the Australian Department of Social Services (n.d.b) as an example, the guidelines strongly warn against using family, friends or close community members as interpreters. It further states that "the use of unqualified or inappropriate interpreters can have serious implications for all parties concerned, particularly where there are legal or health matters involved". The reported behaviours of reception staff members clearly reveal a gap between the policy and the practice in terms of interpreter engagement.

Relatedly, interpreters are hardly regarded as part of a medical team by front desk staff, and this is demonstrated by the identified pattern of not informing interpreters in the case of appointment rescheduling. Many participants said that reception staff members do not bother to call interpreters when changes are made to an appointment. Many interpreters, therefore, end up finding out about rescheduling only after they arrive at hospitals. For example:

> Because sometimes, they cancel the appointment, reschedule the appointment but they didn't let us know so we've been to the appointment and then they tell it. I tried to ring the number but no one answered but they can send an email. It's easy.
>
> (Participant 55, Vietnamese interpreter)

The low recognition of interpreters among front desk staff is demonstrated by failure to contact pre-arranged interpreters for telehealth consultations. In Australia, the government increased subsidisation for telehealth in March 2020 in response to the COVID-19 pandemic, which, in turn, led to a rapid uptake of telehealth services (Savira et al., 2023). Data analysis indicates that despite the increase in telehealth, a lack of understanding about interpreter-enabled telehealth among receptionists serves as a barrier to accessing interpreting services. In the case of face-to-face interpreting, interpreters travel to the site to attend consultations in person, and front desk staff can hardly miss interpreters who are physically there. This is not, however, the case with telehealth, in which interpreters work remotely and are not physically on site. In such cases, front desk staff were reported as often not checking patient files to see if interpreters are booked for NESB patients. Failure to contact pre-arranged interpreter services is demonstrated by the following excerpt:

> The other thing that's happened with COVID unfortunately, at least in our hospital, it's because growing on the phone – we have huge problems with the clinicians not calling us. So they book the session, probably, you know, people in the clinic book and then when it's the time and the patient arrives, they cannot be bothered to call us.
>
> (Participant 21, Italian interpreter)

Conversations with the participants also reveal a lack of training for front desk staff regarding how to work with interpreters. Health care reception staff are required to be trained on health care interpreting including relevant systems and procedures for interpreter arrangement (NSW Health, 2017). The data, however, indicates that this may often not be the case, with many reception staff reportedly having little idea about how to work with interpreters. When booking an interpreter, for example, staff who arrange an interpreter need to enter an exact location for an appointment (e.g., ultrasound department, gynaecology department, etc.) in the booking system, so that interpreters know exactly where to go for the appointment. The participants reported that they are often provided with the generic street address of a hospital, rather than the specific location within the hospital where the appointment takes place. The lack of knowledge about working with interpreters among front desk staff is found to impact an interpreter's ability to arrive on time, as exemplified below:

> She [reception staff member] put the street address of the hospital. In hospital they have many departments, maternity, therapy, yeah. So, it's training for the receptionist staff, the administration staff how to work with interpreters to make the most of the service for them and the interpreter and the client.
>
> (Participant 26, Spanish interpreter)

It bears noting that the low recognition of interpreters among front desk staff occurs within the context of power differentials between frontline staff and interpreters. While reception staff hold lower professional status compared with other health care practitioners (hereafter 'HCPs') such as doctors (Vassy, 2001), they are more powerful than interpreters thanks to their insider status. The participants reported that if reception staff complain about a certain interpreter, there is a high chance that the interpreter may not be asked again. Power differentials tend to be strengthened within the monolingual institutional environment in which interpreters have been traditionally looked down upon (see Section 3.3). The normalisation of disregard for interpreters can be exemplified by the experiences of the participants who have been engaged in the profession for a long time. Taking Participant 4, a Farsi interpreter of over 20 years of experience, as an example, she reported frequent poor treatment by front desk staff during her career. This interpreter has, however, put up with poor treatment due to power asymmetries, as exemplified below:

> So, it's from the beginning. Even people who come across them as receptionists, anybody, because they are so snappy. They are, some are nice, yes, but we should not rely on the fact that this person is nice or is having a nice day rather than this is what should be done. As an interpreter you're vulnerable too, because if you point out these things, they very easily go ahead and they sort of say, we don't want this interpreter anymore.

Data analysis reveals that it is not just interpreters who are disrespected; NESB migrants are sometimes treated poorly too. The participants shared their observations of how NESB migrants are treated as deficient and ignorant others by reception staff. The analysis identifies English monolingualism as a key reason for this reported lack of respect for NESB patients. It was reported that some front desk staff are unwelcoming and rude with patients not fluent in English. Biases against NESB migrants as people of low class are exemplified by the following narrative from Participant 62, a Bosnian interpreter:

> But, you know, just the approach. I think they are the first face there, they should be very nice, very kind, welcoming, at least decent, try your best. But sometimes they look at – not us as interpreters, but the patients, and somehow you feel it, like down, like they are lower class, which is very wrong. Very often at the doctors, they are older people, and in our culture, we really respect older people. You can't treat them that way, raising your voice, stopping them, telling them what to do, it's not nice.

While the class-based dimension of English monolingualism relating to interpreters is not explicitly evident in the data, the common alignment of interpreters with minority patients raises the question of how interpreters are unlikely to be immune to the same biases. The next section examines this question by focusing on how interpreters are treated by doctors.

5.3 Provider perception: interpreters as translation machines

This section examines how interpreters are perceived and treated by doctors in both face-to-face and telephone interpreting contexts.

5.3.1 Face-to-face interpreting

When asked about general experiences of working with doctors, the participants reported both positive and negative aspects of work relations. As for the positive aspects, one-third of the participants expressed satisfaction with working with doctors, pointing out overall improvement in terms of doctors' awareness of interpreting and ability to work with interpreters over the years. Those participants who have been engaged in interpreting for a long time reported that many more HCPs are experienced in working with interpreters than before. Taking Participant 44, a Cantonese interpreter with 23 years of interpreting experience, as an example, the interpreter reported positive changes which contrasted her past experiences:

It's better now than, say, five, ten years ago, even. Yes, I feel that it is better. They're more tolerant of us, and more understanding of what our role is. Whereas before, they just think we're like a person that's holding the other patient's hand, rather than...

While this represents a constructive step in interpreter-provider relations, it is worth paying attention to the participant's choice of "tolerant" to describe the interaction. That expression indicates short-of-full willingness to accept interpreters as legitimate members of a health care team. Issues relating to professional acceptance were, indeed, reported by many participants. In particular, the common use of lay people as interpreters was pointed out as a primary source of dissatisfaction among interpreters in working with doctors. The participants reported that if a patient is accompanied by an English-speaking family member, a doctor would usually prefer to have the bilingual person as an interpreter even when an interpreter is arranged. If a patient can speak English, doctors generally preferred to communicate with the patient directly, rather than going through the interpreter. In such cases, the participants said they would be told that their service is no longer needed or to stay as a 'back-up' in case the patient is unable to cope with the ensuing communications.

Relatedly, the old practice of using any bilingual as interpreters is found to be common among doctors (see Sections 3.3 and 3.4 for details). Be it a nurse, administrative staff or a cleaner, doctors who usually run behind schedule would take whoever is immediately available as an interpreter, rather than trying to arrange for a professional interpreter to attend. For example:

Sometimes they will get a cleaner, and they will say to the cleaner, she speaks Greek, just go and get her. I said no, you can't do that, because you are supposed to get a health care professional, or an accredited interpreter, actually, to interpret for you, and bla-bla-bla. But the doctors, they always think they are the only one who is busy. They always think they are the only ones that don't have time.

(Participant 13, Cantonese interpreter)

The pattern of seeing interpreters as easily replaceable by anyone who speaks more than one language illustrates doctors' disregard of bilingualism as a specialised skill. This reduced view of bilingualism and interpreting is identified as impacting on interpreters' abilities to work professionally. This is evident in the narratives of the other two-thirds of the participants who expressed general dissatisfaction with their work relations with doctors. Data analysis indicates that the most common pattern of behaviours which impacts interpreting is doctors' treatment of interpreters as translation machines, rather than genuine human language experts.

A key indicator of the mechanistic view of interpreters is the reported provider beliefs that interpreters can interpret everything no matter how long, fast-spoken and complicated messages are. According to the participants, some doctors do not even pause to allow time for interpreters to interpret, seeing interpreters as an automatic channel through which their talk can be simultaneously converted to the patient's language. While simultaneous interpreting allows the speaker's messages to be transferred to the client almost at the same time as the speaker utters them, it requires specialised interpreting equipment (e.g., headphones, microphones, etc.). Without special interpreting devices, interpreters are unable to deliver doctors' messages simultaneously. Many doctors are, however, reported to have little understanding about the workings of interpreting and associated challenges, as exemplified below:

> They [doctors] don't know. They think that they can talk and we have to talk together. Simultaneous interpreting won't work when you are at the clinic.
>
> (Participant 30, Arabic interpreter)

The reported tendency to see interpreters as machines is found to be particularly problematic when interpreters try to meet their own professional standards at work. Taking professional ethics as an example, interpreters and translators in Australia are bound by the Code of Ethics, which sets relevant principles for language professionals in Australia (see Australian Institute of Interpreters and Translators, 2012). For interpreters, nine key tenets must be observed in professional practice, including confidentiality, competence, impartiality, accuracy and clarity of role boundaries. Accuracy is generally regarded as the most important professional tenet for interpreters, and the code provides specific guidelines on how to ensure accuracy. Where messages are unclear to the interpreter, for example, the code recommends that "the interpreter asks for repetition, rephrasing or explanation, informing all participants of what is happening" (p. 14). If the interpreter follows this guideline, however, doctors who see interpreters as machines reportedly do not understand why repetition is necessary and do not respond well to such requests. For example:

> But, I guess, that is the nature of the industry so to speak. That's what I thought so. I just don't want to keep telling them [doctors], can you please slow down a bit? If I continue saying that they might at some point get, not angry, but quite upset or they also can be interrupted. So, the professional usually also has to concentrate on what they have to

> do and what should be done within the limited hours, but if their own task is limited or interrupted by the interpreter, because the interpreter is not their main purpose in that scene so to speak. So, I try not to stop or interrupt them too much within the session.
>
> (Participant 6, Korean interpreter)

In addition to managing interactions with doctors, the participants are, at the same time, expected to ensure that NESB patients have understood what has been interpreted. Communication in hospitals tends to be complex due to domain-specific terminologies, and the participants reported that many NESB patients have trouble understanding medical terms. If patients ask for clarification of unfamiliar medical concepts, some doctors were reported as becoming upset at the interpreter who, in their view, has failed to properly deliver messages to the patient. The mechanistic perspective of interpreters, who have to make *everything* understood regardless of patients' capacity to understand the often-complex nature of medical communication, is exemplified by the following narrative:

> Sometimes I find that when the patient doesn't understand a particular medical jargon, particular medical term, and I put it back to the doctor because it's not up to me to explain it or make it easier for them or simpler. It's up to the doctor to explain it. It doesn't go down too well so they say, oh, this is how it is, that's what it is, just tell them what I've told you and I have to tell them. Yeah, and I'm sure that the patient can gather from the doctor's body language and I can gather that they're just not happy about it. I tell the patient, you know, this is what the doctor said, and they say, how are we to understand it, and then the doctor sort of, some of them show a bit of temper. They say, just tell them, so I get this quite a bit, just tell them what I've said, and I just tell them what they've said.
>
> (Participant 22, Arabic interpreter)

It is worth noting how the reported view of interpreters as machines and associated communication problems are compounded by doctors' attitudes to NESB patients. The participants reported that certain doctors see NESB patients as problems and are disrespectful. The reported issue is in line with the recent survey on patient experiences with Australian health care (Zurynski et al., 2022). According to the survey, 23.5 per cent of respondents reported being discriminated against or disrespected when trying to access health care services. Importantly, those respondents were significantly more likely to speak a language other than English at home. While negative experiences are not detailed in the survey, analysis of the data provides a glimpse into doctors' biases against patients not proficient in English.

Data analysis does indicate the doctors' tendency to see NESB patients as difficult and uncooperative. It further indicates the general pattern of attributing any unusual patient behaviours to ethnic stereotypes. This is exemplified by the experiences of Participant 5, a Japanese interpreter. When working as an in-house interpreter for a clinic which had many Japanese patients, the interpreter often encountered doctors who became frustrated at Japanese patients who, in their views, were not willing to cooperate. According to the interpreter, many patients had no prior experience in working with interpreters and were, therefore, unsure about what to do in interpreter-mediated consultations. Due to the lack of experience with working with interpreters, Japanese patients reportedly hesitated in answering questions from doctors, which, in turn, slowed down communications. These types of behaviours were, however, seen as a peculiar ethnic trait, i.e., being cautious or suspicious, by doctors who became impatient with those 'patients unwilling to talk'. For example:

> When I started working in the medical centre, unfortunately I witnessed some of the doctors got frustrated with the Japanese patients. I would have to say that that wasn't professional and you know, patient wasn't happy in the end. That's not something that I would like to achieve [...] Even though they are speaking Japanese but because seeing an Australian doctor, even with an interpreter, because talking through interpreter is not something they're used to. So, they might need more time to express their feelings and so on.
>
> (Participant 5, Japanese interpreter)

The report is a *déjà vu* of ethnic stereotypes prevalent in Australian hospitals in the past (see Section 3.3). NESB patients were commonly discriminated against by HCPs due to the stereotypes which saw them as inadequate, different and difficult. Data analysis reveals that the historical pattern of biases against NESB patients is still present within contemporary hospitals and such biases are to do with patient inability to speak English. In English-monolingual Australian hospitals, speaking English is only natural and those who are unable to perform that natural act are reported as being seen to be deficient. The language biases against NESB patients are demonstrated by the following conversation with Participant 47, a Punjabi interpreter:

> Interpreter: Not rude to the interpreter so to speak, but rude to the patient and they consider the patient as sub-human because they can't speak their language.

> Researcher: How can you tell?
>
> Interpreter: Body language. If you're talking to me on the phone, I can't see your face, I can't see you, you can say anything you like. But once I'm present, I can see you when you're talking to me, your eyes, your body language, you shout louder than your words.

The identified disrespect for NESB patients highlights how monolingual biases are tied to racial and class biases, a tripartite interplay which has long operated in Australian health care (see Chapter 3 for details). It indicates that NESB patients are still subject to linguistic, class and racial biases, and those biases are found to affect interpreters' work. The participants reported experiencing internal conflicts when HCPs said things that were rude and inappropriate to NESB patients. While interpreters are expected to deliver everything, the participants said that they worry about the potential impact of relaying targeted comments on patients. As such, many find it difficult to interpret words directed against patients:

> Sometimes doctors, they would say, he has been stubborn or he didn't listen or something like that. I would tell the doctor, I'm sorry, I have to tell the patient everything. If you don't want me to tell them, don't say it.
>
> (Participant 26, Spanish interpreter)

It was reported that interpreters' dilemmas tend to go unnoticed in an environment in which they are regarded as independent translation machines devoid of feelings and uninterrupted by external factors. Importantly, the identified view of interpreters as machines is found to impact their morale at work. The participants expressed frustration at the ways in which interpreters are treated as invisible, with doctors failing to acknowledge their presence. When interpreters are in the same physical space for face-to-face interpreting, it was reported that many doctors do not bother to extend basic greetings such as saying 'hello'. Being treated as invisible equates to being unimportant. In response, some participants developed professional strategies to overcome a sense of professional identity crisis, and reported them in the interviews. According to Participant 41, a Burmese interpreter, for example, she never fails to wear her interpreter's badge, which, in her own words, helps her to "feel a bit more confident".

While such micro strategies may help protect an interpreter's professional dignity, the view of interpreters as machines may become even more reinforced in certain interpreting contexts. The next section addresses this very question by focusing on telephone interpreting.

5.3.2 Telephone interpreting

In Australia, telehealth is delivered through various means, by telephones, videos and health apps. Among those, telephone interpreting is the most common type of telehealth due to the general availability of and familiarity with the use of telephones (Cho, 2023). At the time of the interviews in the first half of 2022, telephone interpreting was reported as outweighing face-to-face interpreting due to the nationwide lockdowns following the outbreak of COVID-19.

Despite its widespread use, however, telephone interpreting was found to be less preferred than face-to-face interpreting by the participants. They reported that telephone interpreting is affected by various issues including poor reception, signal dropping and cutting-off. These problems are found to commonly occur in the case of telephone interpreting platforms operated by language service providers (LSPs). Depending on assignments, interpreters and other parties are required to log into a designated system for LSP-enabled telephone interpreting, rather than using their own phones for consultations. The quality of telephone interpreting on these systems is said to be very poor, causing frequent interruptions to communication. For example:

> It virtually happened with 80 per cent of the call. In the middle, I can't hear the professional or the professional can't hear me. Or it just dropped out. I call the agency to give feedback and they say, yeah, we're aware of the problem. Many interpreters say the same. So, that's when I know, oh yes. So, each agency has their own line.
>
> (Participant 15, Vietnamese interpreter)

Another challenge associated with telephone interpreting is a lack of opportunities to build rapport with other communication parties, particularly NESB patients. In face-to-face interpreting, there are usually opportunities to break the ice between the interpreter and the patient. For example, interpreters can use friendly gestures such as smiles or may have a short chat with the patient in the waiting room (see Cho, 2021). In telephone interpreting, however, these opportunities are not available and interpreters' inability to see is reported to affect rapport building. Combined with the sound issues, telephone interpreting is said to be a lot more challenging than face-to-face interpreting:

> When you're face-to-face, you build a rapport. I mean, body language helps a lot. While over the phone, you feel that you're so distant from them, and sometimes there's disruptions, sometimes the voice is not

> clear. You face all these problems. Like I'd rather travel one hour [to a hospital], rather than interpret over the phone.
>
> (Participant 54, Arabic interpreter)

Data analysis indicates that the problems associated with telephone interpreting are compounded by the identified tendency of HCPs to see interpreters as translation machines. Analysis of the data shows four common challenges that interpreters encounter in relation to the dominant view of interpreters as translation machines (see also Cho, 2023).

First, the mechanistic view of interpreters is identified as a primary cause for the lack of information provided to telephone interpreters prior to consultations. Various guidelines on working with interpreters in Australia recommend that interpreters be briefed by doctors on the nature of a consultation, particularly in sensitive cases such as domestic violence (see NSW Health, 2017; Victoria Department of Health and Human Services, 2017 for example). Pre-interview briefing is, however, reportedly rare due to the strong provider view of interpreters as machines who can interpret anything and everything without being given prior information. While the lack of briefing affects face-to-face interpreting too, this type of interpreting enables prior interactions between the interpreter and the patient in the waiting room during which the interpreter may obtain useful information for an upcoming consultation. In contrast, many telephone interpreting assignments are said to be on-demand, with whoever is available for a given assignment asked to interpret straight away.

A lack of briefing is reported to significantly compromise interpreters' abilities to manage communication in the case of follow-up consultations. In these, other parties have a shared history, while the interpreter does not. As conversations often resume from where they left off in the previous consultation, it is generally difficult for the interpreter to follow without prior information. Theoretically speaking, interpreters may ask for clarifications, yet being physically invisible is reported to significantly limit the interpreter's capacity to catch the right moment to intervene. Such challenges were, however, said to be not properly understood by doctors who tend to treat briefing as irrelevant to interpreting. For example:

> A lot of the time, the phone interpreting is difficult and we have no idea what we're talking about until we pick up the phone. Sometimes they start talking, and we don't even know, we don't get any briefing, they just start talking, and we don't even know what they're here to talk about until we're starting to get into what they say, then we kind of have some idea. So, that's a hard time, where we don't get any briefing.
>
> (Participant 27, Thai interpreter)

A second challenge is that interaction management is harder in telephone interpreting, compared with face-to-face interpreting. The participants said that some NESB patients see interpreting as an opportunity to express themselves freely and end up speaking at length in interpreter-mediated consultations. As these individuals are unable to express their ideas in English in their daily lives, they "pour out", in the expression of Participant 31, a Korean interpreter, what they want to say when they have an interpreter speaking on their behalf. In face-to-face interpreting, interpreters can cut in by sending verbal or bodily signals (e.g., raising hands), which is, however, not available in the case of telephone interpreting.

The participants reported that doctors often speak at length too. As discussed in the previous section, doctors often do not have adequate knowledge about how interpreting works and tend to believe that interpreters can interpret everything, no matter how long the messages are. According to the participants, they are usually very careful not to upset doctors when they try to cut in, yet it is extremely difficult to work out the right moment to do so in telephone interpreting. Challenges caused by the mechanistic view of interpreting among doctors are described in the following narrative:

> They [doctors] can't go on explaining something for five or 10 minutes, so they have to try and have some portions or I don't know, one or two minutes, but not to go on for ages because obviously the interpreter's memory may be good but, yeah. It's not worth the risk of missing something out because he's explained something for the last 10 minutes.
>
> (Participant 51, Italian interpreter)

Third, HCP perceptions of interpreters as machines render telephone interpreters' inability to see the parties as irrelevant to interpreting. Challenges relating to a lack of visual cues are reported to vary. In cases where visual aids (e.g., X-rays) are employed for communication, interpreters who are unable to see are significantly constrained in their capacity to follow conversations. It was also said to be challenging to work out a communicative context, which is vital to an interpreter's abilities to perform work satisfactorily. In the case of multi-party phone conferences, the participants reported that it is extremely difficult for interpreters (who are usually not briefed) to determine who is involved in the communication and what is being discussed. As interpreters are unable to see for themselves, they have trouble determining whether parties have finished talking. This often leads to speaking before others have finished, causing awkwardness, restarts and repetitions.

Interpreting challenges associated with the inability to see what is going on are found to be compounded in assignments involving elderly

NESB patients. The participants reported that older people are generally unfamiliar with telephone interpreting and some elderly patients even mistake interpreters for doctors. Many do not know how to manage communications through interpreters and generally find telephone interpreting confusing. As such, telephone interpreting for elderly people requires collaboration from HCPs who are in a better position to help elderly patients through being in the same space with them. The onus is, however, often placed on the interpreters, with doctors tending to treat communication as interpreters' sole responsibilities. For example:

> In telephone interpreting, I might ask them [elderly NESB patients] more than the doctor would actually say. If the doctor say, in which part of your body are you experiencing more pain or something? They could be saying leg but not actually saying it. It could be they're pointing to it while talking about it. So when interpreting, I might say, please don't point to it or something like that, or please tell me exactly where it is or something like that simply because it's telephone interpreting. Like I said, old people, they don't realise sometimes they're on the phone or on the video. They just think you're seeing them.
>
> (Participant 32, Indonesian interpreter)

Relatedly, the inability to see in person makes it difficult for interpreters to work out whether patients have understood messages. In face-to-face communication, clues such as nodding or facial expressions reveal a patient's understanding. As such signals are completely absent in telephone interpreting, however, the participants expressed concerns that NESB patients might be inadvertently left out. The nature of such challenges is, however, often not understood by doctors who tend to believe that interpreters can deliver everything even when communicative conditions are not favourable. For example:

> Sometimes maybe, like I was not physically there so sometimes when other professionals suddenly came in, I think, oh no, I thought they were talking to the patient. So, I couldn't see so I was not able to know what happened. So, whenever they speak, I say, sorry, I'm not a machine, I'm not able to remember all of what you said. Because obviously they didn't stop because that was a constant conversation. I say, excuse me, are you able to stop a little bit, I think I need some time to translate to the patient.
>
> (Participant 49, Cantonese interpreter)

In a final challenge, data analysis indicates that sound issues which are particularly prominent in telephone interpreting tend to be dismissed by HCPs due to the dominant provider perception of interpreters as machines. In addition to the sound problems discussed at the beginning of the section, sound issues can exacerbate the situation in emergency departments. Various factors are reported to impact sound quality during telephone interpreting such as screaming from patients in distress, hospital staff running around, document shuffling and people talking loudly. The inadequate quality of sound in these cases is exemplified below:

> Sometimes, especially when the call was from emergency, it was very noisy in the background. Sometimes there were people at the background. They were nurses or different people talking, anesthetists, and I can't even hear them properly.
>
> (Participant 18, Mandarin interpreter)

Sound problems are found to worsen due to the common use of speakerphones. The participants reported that telephones are usually situated far away from parties, which has become more common due to social distancing regulations following the outbreak of the COVID-19 pandemic. Poor sound quality is reported to affect not just interpreters but also patients, particularly people who are hard of hearing (e.g., elderly people). This group of patients with hearing impairment requires specific care to ensure that messages do not get missed. Data analysis, however, identifies the common view of interpreters as machines among HCPs as a significant hindrance to ensuring interpreting accuracy for elderly patients. For example:

> Yeah, well, first of all, as we just said, hearing impairments, so people will have more difficulties to hear you so we really start from the very basic of noisy environment, bad phone lines and people not hearing properly and again, a situation in which the majority you have to go on loudspeaker on the phone in the office of the doctor. It's very, very difficult. Doctors do not understand their patient has to be close to the phone, otherwise we can't hear them
>
> (Participant 21, Italian interpreter)

The findings from this section align with the previous section's discovery of interpreters being viewed as translation machines. It emphasises institutional monolingualism as a primary cause of communication challenges encountered by health care interpreters. As illustrated, interpreting is seen to take place in a vacuum unaffected by external factors which, in fact, significantly impact interpreters' ability to manage communication properly. Not only are those challenges treated as irrelevant to interpreting but their management is seen as the interpreter's sole responsibility. The perception that communication is entirely the interpreter's responsibility goes against the basic tenet of provider-patient communication. According to the Australian Commission on Safety and Quality in Health Care (2016), for example, effective communication and the accurate delivery of information between HCPs and patients are critical to ensuring safe care for patients, and the role of HCPs is highly important to ensuring successful communications in that arena. This is clearly not observed in interpreter-mediated communications.

The identified perception of interpreting as a mechanistic activity among HCPs suggests that NESB patients might be disadvantaged in interpreter-mediated settings. It can be extremely difficult for interpreters to deliver the right messages when they have no knowledge of the communication context, cannot hear, and/or cannot see what is going on. The monolingual way of (not) understanding bilingual communications, therefore, represents not just challenges to interpreters but also to linguistic minorities due to potential access inequity.

5.4 Systemic problems

This section examines problems relating to hospital systems which affect the interpreter's capacity to perform work. Data analysis identifies two major problems: long waiting times for consultations; and an inadequate amount of consultation time for interpreter-mediated communication.

To begin with, the participants pointed to long waiting times as a cause of conflict with HCPs. It was reported that all too often, interpreters (and patients) end up waiting for consultations too long, which, in turn, has a cascading impact on subsequent assignments to which interpreters have been allocated. As interpreters are required to be punctual, long waits were reported to make the participants feel anxious and worrisome. The participants reported that most hospitals do not seem to understand that interpreters have other assignments to attend to and that consultations need to take place at the scheduled time to allow interpreters to move on to their next assignment promptly. During the interviews, the participants expressed feelings of frustration at the lack of institutional understanding about the interpreter's own needs. For example:

> I mean, I can understand the patients, okay, but it's not acceptable that the professionals you work with do not understand things so much and working in hospital. As I say, it's really a waiting game when we do it face to face which is very frustrating and it's not considered the way it should be considered.
>
> (Participant 21, Italian interpreter)

The participants reported that they often need to leave for their next assignment by the time that the consultation gets started. This is found to cause tensions with HCPs, because many do not understand why interpreters have another job, not to mention the long wait as the main culprit behind the problem. It was reported that many HCPs therefore get upset at interpreters who in their views have caused inconvenience to their work. For example:

> Your appointment is 5:30 but it's 7:30 now it's still not your turn, you still haven't been called. Yeah, sometimes we were called into the doctor's consultation room and then it's just five minutes before our booking finishes. Then the doctor they say I haven't finished you know? I haven't finished with this patient how can you leave? This causes some unnecessary tension between interpreters and the doctors.
>
> (Participant 12, Mandarin interpreter)

Data analysis identifies a general tendency to use interpreters at will, most clearly illustrated by the lack of respect for their time. Interpreters are generally expected to stay until HCPs are finished, regardless of interpreters' own work schedules. If interpreters tried to remind HCPs of their need to leave promptly, such requests are found to be generally met with negative responses:

> So, I start interpreting and the doctors go on and on and on and 20 minutes up. So, I gently tell the professional, I'm sorry, I was booked only for 20 minutes. Then almost always the doctors got angry, and they were very rude to me.
>
> (Participant 31, Korean interpreter)

Second, the allocation of standard consultation time to interpreter-assisted communication was reported as another chronic systemic issue which impacts interpreters' capacity. In Australia, a standard single GP consultation is generally 15 minutes, with the initial consultation usually an extended appointment of 30 minutes (Australian Patients Association, 2022). In the case of an interpreter-mediated consultation, communication takes at least double that time, because the interpreter repeats what was said by each party. Interpreter-assisted consultations, therefore, require longer time to ensure full communication. This is, however, found to be hardly the case.

Data analysis indicates that the standard consultation time of 15 minutes is generally allocated to interpreter-mediated consultations. The lack of consultation time impacts interpreters' capacity to do their jobs properly, as HCPs tend to rush to cover everything within a limited time. Some HCPs were reported to cut short interpreting or interrupt in the middle of interpreting. Furthermore, it was reported that most patients do not get to ask everything due to the insufficient amount of time for consultations. This issue is particularly problematic in the case of culturally sensitive topics such as sexual health. Taking sexually transmitted diseases as an example, the participants said that it is a cultural taboo to discuss these things in certain societies (see also Section 6.3.1). As patients with these conditions feel ashamed, it takes time for them to open up and fully discuss their health concerns. The process of 'warm-up' to help patients to feel comfortable is, however, reported to be unfeasible due to the insufficient amount of time for consultations in interpreter-mediated communication. This leads patients to feel frustrated and worried, which, in turn, stresses interpreters, as exemplified in the following:

> So yes, the practitioner, most of the time they are likely to say I do understand that you have a lot of questions but because our time is up, we can arrange a next time. So we can ask more question. What do you think of that? But then the client actually asking questions. No, no, I want my question to be answered today. But then me, I translate it to the practitioner and the practitioner keep saying the same thing that hey, I won't be able to answer it. Please arrange another appointment. Which is good for me as well because I can attend the next job. But then from a client perspective, I can see their frustration. You know they want their answer to be, their question to be answered today. Because this is, look, they're dealing with stigma and we're not too sure about how they are going to make assumption of this diagnosis themselves when they're at home.
>
> (Participant 56, Cambodian interpreter)

Analysis of the data highlights a significant lack of institutional understanding and consideration for interpreter-mediated communications. The very basic need of interpreting, such as requiring at least double the amount of regular consultation time, is found to be not accommodated for health care interpreting. Furthermore, the system is found to be ignorant of interpreters' professional needs, such as enabling them to attend assignments at the scheduled time to allow for timely transitions to their next assignment. These systemic problems are concerning, considering their potential impact on NESB patients. It is fair to ask how NESB patients can receive quality consultations when interpreters have to leave early. It is also fair to ask how NESB patients can receive full consultations when they are technically given only half the time they need. Ultimately, we must question why these problems persist nearly 50 years after the establishment of the Health Care Interpreter Service. The findings highlight that interpreting issues do not just affect interpreters but also impact the linguistic minorities they serve.

5.5 Summary

This chapter has examined how interpreters are perceived and treated in Australian health care institutions at three levels – front desk staff, doctors and hospital systems. It reveals that interpreting is generally under-appreciated at all levels of health care institutions. The findings highlight that interpreting challenges are attributable to institutional monolingualism characterised by a significant lack of understanding and consideration of the distinctive nature and needs of interpreting. There are three important findings related to institutional monolingualism.

First, the findings highlight that interpreting tends to be poorly understood and that interpreters are treated with disrespect by front desk staff. The findings reveal that many reception staff are not trained to work with interpreters, despite the recommendations from relevant guidelines, which, in turn, affects the ways interpreters perform their jobs. Furthermore, interpreters are found to be treated with little professional respect due to the general perception of interpreting as a job which any bilingual can perform. Importantly, the findings show the racial and class-based biases of English monolingualism against NESB patients who tend to be subject to discrimination within the traditionally monolingual milieu of health care institutions. These discoveries are in line with the historical pattern of English monolingualism in Australian health care (see Sections 3.3 and 3.4 for details), highlighting the strong workings of institutional monolingualism within contemporary Australian hospitals.

Second, the poor perception and treatment of interpreters are found to be the case with doctors too, as illustrated by the identified view of interpreters as translation machines. Rather than accepted as legitimate professionals, interpreters are seen as robots who need to be self-sufficient and self-responsible for anything to do with communication. Similar to the previously mentioned findings (see Section 3.3), NESB patients are found to be subject to racial and class biases embedded in English monolingualism in their interactions with doctors. Once again, the findings emphasise institutional monolingualism as the primary cause of communication problems experienced by interpreters. This book questions how and why the inadequate understanding of interpreting continues after almost half a century since health care interpreting was introduced. As discussed in Chapter 3, interpreting was not properly understood among HCPs at its start, with interpreters struggling to be accepted as professional equals in the monolingual institutional milieu. The discovery of the same problems within hospitals today indicates that Australian health care remains fundamentally monolingual, failing to understand the specific nature and needs of bilingual communications.

Third, institutional monolingualism is found to affect interpreters at a systemic level too. The problems relating to long wait-times and inadequate consultation times highlight the institutional ignorance of interpreting and, by extension, NESB patients. Problems such as long waits are entirely addressable, if hospitals give priority to interpreter-assisted consultations when an appointment is made. The same goes for the allocation of standard consultation time to interpreter-mediated sessions. Analysis shows that little institutional consideration has been given to the problems experienced by interpreters, which, once again, emphasises the monolingual way of not understanding the specific nature of bilingual communication. Above all, it is concerning that NESB patients might be disadvantaged due to the inadequate consideration given to interpreting services in hospitals.

Taken together, the findings highlight the normalisation of poor perceptions and treatment of health care interpreting and interpreters within contemporary Australian health care institutions. Many of the problems identified in this chapter are similar to the issues reported by the first health care interpreters many years ago (see Section 3.3). The resemblance between the problems back then and the problems now points to a huge gap between the system, which is regarded as a model, and the reality of interpreters struggling under the system characterised by institutional monolingualism. It emphasises the monolingual approach to interpreting as the most significant obstacle to the development of health care interpreting.

The findings are particularly important when considering the possibility that the poor treatment of interpreters may translate into poorer health outcomes for NESB patients. The identified pattern of ignorance of interpreting problems among HCPs raises concerns about the quality of communication for linguistic minorities. While ignoring communication issues which may potentially impact the health of patients would undoubtedly be unacceptable, the very fact that this pattern of behaviours continues in interpreter-mediated consultations reveals conscious or unconscious biases against NESB patients. For example, would institutions ask any bilingual to interpret for someone who does not speak English well yet is in a powerful position? The answer would probably be no. The chapter reveals that institutional monolingualism is strongly tied to not only linguistic but also racial and class biases, which have long characterised Australian health care. This may explain why progress has been so slow in raising awareness of interpreting as a key to enhancing access, equity and social participation for linguistic minorities.

References

Au, M., Preston, R., Ray, R. A., & Davis, M. (2021). Refugee healthcare perceptions in regional northern Australia: Transition through engagement, access, trust, privacy, the old, and the new. *Australian Journal of Primary Health*, *27*(5), 382–390. https://doi.org/10.1071/PY20265

Australian Commission on Safety and Quality in Health Care. (2016). *Patient-Clinician Communication in Hospitals*. www.safetyandquality.gov.au/sites/default/files/migrated/Information-sheet-for-healthcare-providers-Improving-patient-clinician-communication.pdf

Australian Institute of Interpreters and Translators. (2012). *AUSIT Code of Ethics and Code of Conduct*. https://ausit.org/wp-content/uploads/2024/09/AUSIT-Code-of-Ethics-and-Code-of-Conduct.pdf

Australian Patients Association. (2022). *Doctor Consultations*. www.patients.org.au/doctor-consultations/

Bayram, C., Ryan, R., Harrison, C., Gardiner, J., Bailes, M. J., Obeyesekere, N., ... & Britt, H. (2016). Consultations conducted in languages other than English in Australian general practice. *Australian Family Physician*, *45*(1–2), 9–13.

Bird, S. (2010). Failure to use an interpreter. *Australian Family Physician*, *39*(4), 241–242.

Bischoff, A. (2020). The evolution of a healthcare interpreting service mapped against the bilingual health communication model: A historical qualitative case study. *Public Health Reviews*, *41*(19), 1–25. https://doi.org/10.1186/s40985-020-00123-8

Blay, N., Ioannou, S., Seremetkoska, M., Morris, J., Holters, G., Thomas, V., & Bronwyn, E. (2018). Healthcare interpreter utilisation: Analysis of health administrative data. *BMC Health Services Research*, *18*, 1–6. https://doi.org/10.1186/s12913-018-3135-5

Cheng, J. H., Wang, C., Jhaveri, V., Morrow, E., Li, S. T. T., & Rosenthal, J. L. (2021). Health care provider practices and perceptions during family-centered rounds with limited English-proficient families. *Academic Pediatrics*, *21*(7), 1223–1229. https://doi.org/10.1016/j.acap.2020.12.010

Cho, J. (2021). *Intercultural communication in interpreting: Power and choices*. Routledge. https://doi.org/10.4324/9781003179993

Cho, J. (2023). Interpreters as translation machines: Telephone interpreting challenges as awareness problems. *Qualitative Health Research*, *33*(12), 1037–1048. https://doi.org/10.1177/10497323231191712

Collyer, F. M., Willis, K. F., & Lewis, S. (2017). Gatekeepers in the healthcare sector: Knowledge and Bourdieu's concept of field. *Social Science & Medicine*, *186*, 96–103. https://doi.org/10.1016/j.socscimed.2017.06.004

Department of Social Services. (n.d.a). *Doctors Priority Line*. www.materonline.org.au/MaterOnline/media/materonline/PDFs/Doctors-Priority-Line-DSS-Information-Brochure.pdf

Department of Social Services. (n.d.b). *Using Interpreters and Family Safety*. www.dss.gov.au/sites/default/files/documents/12_2019/fact-sheet-using-interpreters-and-family-safety-updated-17-december-2019.pdf

Garrett, P. (2009). Healthcare interpreter policy: Policy determinants and current issues in the Australian context. *Translation & Interpreting: The International Journal of Translation and Interpreting Research*, *1*(2), 44–54.

Health Care Interpreter Service. (n.d.). *Do you need an interpreter?*. www.file:///C:/Users/midan/Downloads/ABC%20Tool%20for%20Assessing%20the%20Need%20for%20an%20Interpreter.pdf

Migrant & Refugee Health Partnership. (2020). *Interpreter Engagement in General Practice in Australia*. https://culturaldiversityhealth.org.au/wp-content/uploads/2020/06/Interpreter-Engagement-in-General-Practice-in-Australia.pdf

NSW Health. (2017). *Interpreters – Standard Procedures for Working with Health Care Interpreters*. www1.health.nsw.gov.au/pds/ActivePDSDocuments/PD2017_044.pdf

Phillips, C. B., & Travaglia, J. (2011). Low levels of uptake of free interpreters by Australian doctors in private practice: Secondary analysis of national data. *Australian Health Review*, *35*(4), 475–479. https://doi.org/10.1071/AH10900

Quick, B. E. (2024). *How are language barriers bridged in hospitals?: A systematic review* [Master's dissertation, Macquarie University]. https://doi.org/10.25949/25294231.v1

Savira, F., Orellana, L., Hensher, M., Gao, L., Sanigorski, A., Mc Namara, K., ... & Peeters, A. (2023). Use of general practitioner telehealth services during the COVID-19 pandemic in regional Victoria, Australia: Retrospective analysis. *Journal of Medical Internet Research*, *25*, e39384. https://doi.org/10.2196/39384

Vassy, C. (2001). Categorisation and micro-rationing: Access to care in a French emergency department. *Sociology of Health & Illness*, *23*(5), 615–632. https://doi.org/10.1111/1467-9566.00268

Victoria Department of Health and Human Services. (2017). *Language Services Policy*. www.dhhs.vic.gov.au/ publications/language-services-policy-and-guidelines

Zurynski, Y., Ellis, L. A., Dammery, G., Smith, C. L., Halim, N., Ansell, J., Gillespie, J., Caffery, L., Vitangcol, K., Wells, L., & Braithwaite, J. (2022). *The Voice of Australian Health Consumers: The 2021 Australian Health Consumer Sentiment Survey. Report prepared for the Consumers Health Forum of Australia*. https://chf.org.au/sites/default/files/pchss_consumersentimentsurveyreport_final3.pdf

6 Individual responses to monolingualism

6.1 Why do interpreters stay in the field?

One puzzle which constantly arose during the interviews was why the participants adhered to the profession of interpreting, despite the problems already examined and general under-appreciation of interpreting identified. In trying to address the puzzle, this chapter specifically looks at why the participants stay in the field through the concept of *illusio* proposed by Bourdieu (1998; see also Bourdieu & Wacquant, 1992). The notion of *illusio* refers to the adherence and commitment of agents or players to their fields and individual investment in the stakes of the game. According to Bourdieu:

> Every social field ... tends to require those entering it to have the relationship to the field that I call *illusio*. They may want to overturn the relations of force within the field, but for that very reason, they grant recognition to the stakes, they are not indifferent. Wanting to undertake a revolution in a field is to accord the essential of what the field tacitly demands, namely that it is important, that the game played is sufficiently important for one to want to undertake a revolution in it.
>
> (Bourdieu, 1998, p. 78)

Bourdieu further argues that "Players agree, by the mere fact of playing, and not by way of a 'contract', that the game is worth playing, that it is 'worth the candle', and this collusion is the very basis of their competition" (Bourdieu & Wacquant, 1992, p. 98, emphasis in original). As a relatively under-used Bourdieusian theory, *illusio* has received attention in recent years from scholars interested in individual career aspirations and player interactions with the field (see Connolly et al., 2016; Lupu & Empson, 2015; Nölleke et al., 2022). It is through *illusio* or the acceptance of the fundamental premise that the game is worth being serious about that players invest in the stakes, which may vary by individual. While playing

DOI: 10.4324/9781032614854-6

the game, however, players may experience a gap between aspirations and realities at which they feel displaced and experience the shattering of *illusio* (see Colley, 2012). Only a handful of works on *illusio* relate to interpreting, and the extant studies approach *illusio* from both personal and professional angles. At the professional level, *illusio* relates to interpreter interactions with professional norms, i.e., local code of conduct. At the personal level, *illusio* refers to an individual's commitment to helping vulnerable populations to ensure equitable access.

Colley and Guéry (2015) explore both dimensions of *illusio* in the case of the professional experiences of public service interpreters (PSIs) in the U.K. As for interpreters' interactions with the local code of conduct, the research identifies three types of *illusio*. These include strict individual adherence to the norm, modified adoptions of the norm, and conflicts between the norm's requirements and requests from established professionals who hold more power than interpreters (e.g., doctors and lawyers). The study finds that interpreters generally try to observe the Code of Conduct, which requires them to stay strictly neutral and impartial whilst delivering accurate and excellent linguistic output. Conflicts arise, however, when interpreters are forced to step out of their prescribed professional roles, such as when they are asked to provide emotional support for migrant clients. While these expectations may align with the personal-level *illusio* of helping the vulnerable, their practice goes against the professional norms, leading many to feel 'caught' in the field.

The personal dimension of *illusio* is also explored in research on PSIs from refugee backgrounds working for Syrian refugees in Turkey (Ulaş & Gündüz, 2020). The study specifically investigates interpreters' motivations that lie behind the profession at large and also individually held values attached to interpreting. Having language skills is identified as one common motivation, yet the study identifies a significant sense of satisfaction from helping refugees from the same ethnic background as a strong driver behind interpreter development of 'feel for the game'. While the income generated from the profession was found to be low, economic capital was reported to be not the top priority of those interpreters; it was the moral dimension of the job and a sense of humanity that kept them engaged in the field.

This chapter builds on the existing body of work to examine the dual dimensions of *illusio* – personal aspirations and professional norms experienced by health care interpreters in Australia. It specifically investigates how individually held beliefs in interpreting influence the ways in which interpreters navigate professional norms within the monolingual milieu of Australian health care institutions. The next section looks at the first question of why interpreters do what they do in relation to individual meanings attached to interpreting.

6.2 It is still worth it

During the interviews, a question of 'do you like interpreting and why?' was asked of the participants at the end of each conversation. Considering the various problems discussed during the interviews, it was assumed that many would say no. The surprising response of a majority was that they liked interpreting and wanted to continue to be engaged in the field. Data analysis indicates four primary reasons behind the participants' commitment to the field: love for language; intellectual stimulation; professional dynamism; and helping those in need.

To begin with, many participants reported their love for language as a primary reason behind their beliefs in the worthiness of staying in the field. Responses ranged from enjoyment of language learning, interest in linguistics, to personal attachment to the mother tongue. For this group of participants, interpreting represents an ideal space in which they can continue to do what they truly enjoy. While the market treatment of bilingualism as a non-skill was found to frustrate many participants (see Chapter 4), it does not entirely negate the amount of satisfaction they derive from interpreting. Many were willing to compromise. For example:

> So, because of that, because one way I could keep in touch with my language. So, from that perspective, it gives me that satisfaction and that's why I said if my employer [from the other full-time job] is paying me more than $100 an hour, why should I accept $40 an hour [for interpreting]. But I'm still willing to accept $60 an hour or something like that.
>
> (Participant 34, Hindi interpreter)

Another driver that led the participants to adhere to the profession relates to interpreting as a source of intellectual stimulation. Due to the nature of interpreting in which each situation covers a new domain, interpreting is said to allow the participants to constantly learn new things, stimulating them intellectually. As expressed by Participant 47, an Urdu interpreter, interpreting is worth it because "every case is different, and you are on your toes, and your senses are heightened at that time when you're listening". Participant 38, a Japanese interpreter, put it this way:

> I like interpreting because it's intellectually stimulating. It's a no end point, like you always have to learn or you always learn new things from any assignment.

Relatedly, the constantly dynamic nature of interpreting was cited as another reason behind the participants' commitment to the field. During the interviews, the participants specifically described interpreting as a profession which enables them to be adventurous. These participants enjoy constant exposure to novelty including meeting new people, going to new places as well as learning new things. The new experiences they have gained from interpreting have, in turn, enriched their life, and for this very reason, the participants reported adhering to the field. For example:

> I like human interaction. I like going to places to – you know it's different every day. I drive a lot every day and I think – I like the combination of you need to be active to a certain degree, but then when you go and sit there your body can sit and rest, but your mind, your brain's working.
>
> (Participant 14, Thai interpreter)

Finally, data analysis identifies satisfaction from helping migrants not fluent in English as the most significant motivation behind staying in the game. As many as 60% of the 67 participants reported deriving a sense of satisfaction from helping people unable to communicate freely. For example, Participant 39, the Italian interpreter who admitted a heightened sense of dissatisfaction with the material conditions of interpreting (see Section 4.3.2), expressed how much she enjoys helping others through interpreting:

> I love interpreting because I really help the communication. I facilitate the communication between people who are usually totally helpless because either they're elderly, but they're also sick. They are in the worst possible situation, and it makes me feel very well when I can see that I help them.

Many participants specifically mentioned feeling proud of making a difference in the lives of marginalised individuals with their bilingual skills. The participants, many of whom were not fluent in English when they first arrived in Australia, understood only too well the impact of communication challenges and feelings of helplessness from their migration journeys. Many participants expressed sympathy for the struggles experienced by NESB migrants, reaffirming their commitment to helping those in need:

> Language is power and if you don't have that access to communication, you will remain a very powerless individual in Australia. I really feel for that because when I came to Australia as a teenager, that's the problem that I faced. I could not express my wishes or could not make decisions properly, because of the language barrier. So, I experienced it, I felt it

> and because I have the skills now, I would like to use that to help those who are in the same situation.
>
> (Participant 31, Korean interpreter)

People who need an interpreter's help are mostly from the same ethnic communities, and ethnic solidarity through giving to community figures prominently in the data analysis. From the perspectives of these community interpreters, centrally involved in day-to-day communication management for NESB populations, the playing field is not even for migrants, particularly for individuals with limited English. A case in point is workers' compensation cases. Elderly migrants from non-English-speaking parts of Europe, many of whom came to Australia as part of Australia's mid-20th century immigration drive (see Section 3.1), might have lived in Australia for a long time, yet many are not fluent in English. They went straight into work areas, which did not require much English. While their English might be sufficient to manage their daily lives, NESB elderly migrants often have trouble expressing themselves in English in adversarial situations such as workers' compensation cases. For example:

> It's not that they don't speak English. Many of them, they work in the factory. They came here on the Monday and they started working in a factory the next day and it was in those days 40, 50 years ago, maybe 30 years ago. Yeah, when we first came, there was plenty of work and so they, their English is really limited. Of course, they can tell you all the names of the tools they use doing formwork for example or in carpentry. But when it comes to this [workers' compensation], particularly when emotions are affected, they cannot explain themselves properly.
>
> (Participant 16, Spanish interpreter)

Analysis of the interview data shows language-related inequalities experienced by NESB populations as a key motivator behind participant commitment to interpreting. The participants saw themselves as fortunate to have bilingual skills, and described interpreting as an obligation to return their good fortune to the vulnerable members of the ethnic communities. Some participants expressed that serving their own communities through interpreting is not a matter of option, but an ethnic duty:

> I look at it as an obligation, as a duty, to anything that I do in the community. You do it because you're obliged to. I'm an older person who's had a lot of luck and good fortune in life. I'm obliged to – I'm obliged. It's an obligation. It's not whether I want to or like to. I'm obliged to contribute to the community.
>
> (Participant 58, Hebrew interpreter)

The same sentiment was echoed by many participants who had a full-time job and were engaged in interpreting part-time. While those participants emphasised the necessity of having a job other than interpreting to make it financially sustainable (see Section 4.4), their primary motivator behind keeping interpreting part-time was not necessarily money but helping others in vulnerable situations. Some interpreters reported sometimes providing free interpreting services to people who could not afford to pay. For example, Participant 45, a Tamil interpreter, reported having not charged clients experiencing financial hardship, saying that she felt sympathy for NESB migrants' struggles. The importance of interpreting as a tool for community service and ethnic empowerment was constantly highlighted during the interviews. For example:

> This is not just for the money, the second, another income. It's also, I do this to support and contribute back to my community what I can. It's because I'm lucky enough to go through the good schooling in Burma, learned both Burmese and English well, so I can do the interpreting and translation. It's my contribution back to the community.
>
> (Participant 43, Burmese interpreter)

The findings highlight strong ties between personal *illusio*, migration and minority status in interpreting. Many participants accepted that the game is worth playing due to their own migrant backgrounds and sympathy for fellow ethnic groups who struggle in Australia. Interpreting is a means of ethnic empowerment, which the participants feel is both responsible and rewarding. Through this *illusio*, interpreters bring their experiences of living as a minority individual to the field, which is yet dominated by established professionals. Having identified interpreting as a moral obligation to help the vulnerable as individual-level *illusio*, the next section examines how personal meanings attached to interpreting intersect with the other type of *illusio* relating to professional norms and institutional monolingualism of Australian hospitals.

6.3 Alone or together? Managing communication problems

This section explores the intersections between personal aspirations, professional requirements and institutional monolingualism when interpreters try to address culture-related communication challenges.

6.3.1 Navigating the field

Our conversations reveal culture as a key source of communication challenges for interpreting. Data analysis identifies various concepts, terms and syndromes that are hard to interpret due to cultural specificity. Table 6.1 lists culture-bound terms which are tricky to interpret, as reported by the participants:

An interpreter's own abilities to manage cultural problems are important, yet equally important is collaboration with established professionals who have the power to dictate the terms of the game (see Cho, 2021, 2023; Colley & Guéry, 2015). As examined extensively in Chapter 5, interpreting is predominantly regarded as a mechanistic activity among HCPs in Australia. This monolingual understanding of interpreting is found to be particularly problematic in the case of communication problems relating to culture.

Data analysis indicates five problems relating to HCP awareness of culture and interpreting. First, it was reported that doctors prioritise Australian cultural norms over the patients' own culture. Second, HCPs tend to look for instant solutions to complex cultural issues which arise in interpreting. Third, many HCPs believe they understand culture and there is no need to learn about cultures other than their own. Fourth, some HCPs do not allow interpreters enough time to explain cultural differences to them and/or patients. Finally, the participants reported that some HCPs do not change after cultural issues are raised by and discussed

Table 6.1 Culture-specific communication problems

Challenges	*Explanations*
The unmentionable	Terms that are culturally feared and believed to reinforce existing conditions through verbalisation (e.g., cancer)
Culture-bound medical syndromes	Conditions that have widespread familiarity in one culture and are non-existent in others
Emotions & feelings	Different ways of describing emotions or feelings across cultures
Gender & sex	Gender- and sex-related terms and topics that are culturally inappropriate to discuss particularly by the other gender
Mental illnesses	Avoidance or denial of mental conditions among patients and family due to cultural stigma attached to mental illness
Newly coined terms	Medical terms that have been recently created and have yet to be familiarised by some cultures (e.g., social distancing)
Systemic differences	Terms and concepts relating to medical systems in one culture which are not familiar to patients from another

with interpreters. Overall, culture was reportedly not taken seriously by many doctors, as exemplified below:

> To me, from my experience, they want to go, go, go and finish it off and get the consent form signed, everything done. With the cultural beliefs, I don't think they care or even ask about it at all.
>
> (Participant 17, Thai interpreter)

The participants expressed that it is stressful dealing with complex cultural problems when working with HCPs who do not understand interpreting and generally treat culture as irrelevant to it:

> It's quite difficult because I tend to be caught in between and squashed like a sandwich as we say.
>
> (Participant 25, Greek interpreter)

Challenges encountered by interpreters are found to be compounded by a lack of clear guidelines on inter-party collaboration relating to communication challenges in interpreting. Taking the Code of Ethics and Code of Conduct for interpreters in Australia as an example, clear role boundaries are drawn, as exemplified by the following requirement: "Practitioners do not, in the course of their interpreting or translation duties, engage in other tasks such as advocacy, guidance or advice" (Australian Institute of Interpreters and Translators, 2012, p. 6). At the same time, the Code recognises that the effective provision of language services is a "shared responsibility" (Australian Institute of Interpreters and Translators, 2012, p. 11). There is, however, little guidance on how interpreters and other parties should work together when communication challenges arise. One exception is Clause 5.4, which stipulates "Where circumstances permit, interpreters and translators ask for repetition, rephrasing or explanation if anything is unclear" (p. 10). This assumes willingness to collaborate from other established players but may not work, considering the identified tendency of HCPs who see interpreters as independent translation robots (see Section 5.3 for details).

The lack of clear rules on how the game should be played identifies interpreting as an ill-defined profession, in which players often experience discordance between expectations and experiences (see Bourdieu, 2000). At the same time, however, the ill-defined nature of the profession may represent possibilities for players to play the game on their own terms by redefining the profession to suit who they are (Bourdieu, 2000). Data analysis identifies that the participants have developed various individual strategies to deal with culture-related communication problems.

Table 6.2 provides the details of the identified strategies.

Table 6.2 Interpreters' strategies

	Independent strategies		*Collaborative strategies involving HCPs*	*Collaborative strategies involving patients*
Norm-oriented strategy	Interpreting everything exactly as it is		Asking HCPs to clarify meanings while informing patients	Asking the patient to clarify meanings while informing HCPs
	Explaining interpreters' roles in advance			
Norm-adjusted strategy	Self-contained strategies	Approximation Avoiding eye contact Borrowing from other language Delivering only the essence Euphemism Highlighting key words Paraphrasing Simplifying terms Substitution Unpacking meanings Using gestures and props Varying tone of voice Watering meanings down	Asking HCPs to simplify complex concepts Explaining to HCPs why the patient fails to understand Pre-discussion with HCPs about tricky cultural issues	
	Open strategies	Stepping in to offer cultural explanations to HCPs		
		Suggesting HCPs hire another interpreter		
Norm-resistant strategy	Sharing interpreters' personal experiences		Suggesting HCPs modify test items (e.g., cognitive assessment for elderly)	
	Taking extra care for patients outside consultations			

Note: The strategies are arranged alphabetically.

Two key factors were used to define these interpreter strategies: i) the degree of adherence to the Code of Conduct or professional *illusio*; ii) the degree of collaboration with other parties. According to the degree of adherence to the Code of Conduct, three categories of strategies emerged: norm-oriented, norm-adjusted and norm-resistant. A norm-oriented strategy refers to the reported tendency to strictly abide by the codified norm by focusing on accuracy and neutrality. The second category, a norm-adjusted strategy, refers to the flexibility which interpreters exercise to deliver culture-specific messages, yet without completely deviating from the rules. Finally, a norm-resistant strategy is one that an interpreter deploys in a given situation in their own way without considering the norm. Identification of the latter strategy is based on a clear breach of the Code, with the breach of role boundaries identified as its most prominent element.

As for the degree of collaboration with other parties, three types of strategies emerge: i) independent strategies or strategies independently employed by interpreters which do not involve other parties; ii) collaborative strategies with HCPs; iii) collaborative strategies with patients, excluding HCPs. As can be seen in Table 6.2, most strategies fall under 'independent strategies', in which interpreters act alone without involving other parties. Table 6.2 also shows that many strategies are concentrated within the category of 'norm-adjusted strategies', which indicates that interpreters exercise flexibility in dealing with communication problems. The following section examines the reported strategies in detail with a focus on rationales behind the adoption of the strategies.

6.3.2 Interpreters' strategies

This section explores the strategies reported by the participants.

6.3.2.1 Norm-oriented strategies

Data analysis indicates that norm-oriented strategies are used independently by interpreters, as well as collaboratively with other parties, including HCPs and patients. As for strategies involving patients, the participants seek clarification from patients regarding any unclear messages, while informing HCPs. This strategy is in line with the Code, which stipulates that "If anything is unclear, the interpreter asks for repetition, rephrasing or explanation, informing all participants of what is happening" (Australian Institute of Interpreters and Translators, 2012, p. 14). The strategy was reported to be useful when unpacking culture-specific health conditions which are not known to HCPs. A good example is *loong*, *tripa* and *baekan*, medical concepts specific to Tibet (Cameron & Namdul, n.d.).

According to Participant 50, a Tibetan interpreter, the concepts represent three primary sources of energies which are believed to affect health conditions among Tibetans (see also Cameron & Namdul, n.d.). It was reported that patients often cite those elements as a health condition, rather than providing specific details about their health, saying 'I have *loong*', for example. In such cases, the interpreter asks the patient to elaborate further on their conditions to capture specific meanings. For example:

> So, all diseases come down to these three groups [*loong*, *tripa* and *baekan*]. It is quite complicated, you know? If a patient says to me, I have *baekan* but then because I have no idea what it is. Then I ask him or her so what is your suffering? Or what is your problem, difficulties, can you explain me in detail? Then the patient explains me in plain language. Yep, yep and then she says, oh, I have stomachache or have this, that and I have digestion problem or some like this. Then it is easier for me to translate it.

The strategy of seeking clarification is found to be used with HCPs too. The participants reported that they ask HCPs to break down the intended meanings of culture-specific terms to ensure accurate interpreting. As an example, 'upset' is commonly used in Australia to describe feelings of worry, unhappiness and/or anger in a collective sense. This word was, however, reportedly non-existent in many cultures in which feelings and emotions are more nuanced. According to the participants, the multiple meanings embedded in 'upset' cannot be condensed into a single word, and translating it, therefore, requires the interpreter to understand how the word is intended to be meant by HCPs. For this reason, interpreters such as Participant 32, an Indonesian interpreter, asked HCPs to explain the exact meaning of 'upset' as intended by them before commencing interpreting. For example:

> I have to ask the doctor whether the doctor was aiming for the patient explaining more about being sad or being angry. It depends. If it's a discussion about depression or stress or if it's a discussion about domestic abuse or something like anger management, depending on what the appointment is, then I have to usually just ask the doctor to verify what emotion he's trying [to get] the patient to convey.

As for the independent strategies, two are identified: i) interpreting everything exactly as it is; ii) explaining interpreters' role in advance. The latter strategy is used to handle requests from parties that exceed the interpreter's role expectations and boundaries; cancer is a good example.

It was reported that cancer is culturally feared in many cultures and people in those cultures avoid saying the word 'cancer' for fear that verbalising it would strengthen the condition (see Table 6.1). For example, patients from Arabic-speaking countries tend to use 'the c-word' rather than say 'cancer', according to Participant 22, an Arabic interpreter. Attitudes to cancer, however, differ significantly in Australia in which the patient's right to know is prioritised (Cho, 2021). Cultural differences relating to cancer are exemplified below:

> This is the first time the patient had got the results of the testing and then the doctor is straight in, you're stage four cancer, there is no treatment available unless it is that kind. (Participant 1, Japanese interpreter)

The Australian approach to cancer is found to be too confronting to many NESB patients and families. The participants reported that families present at consultations often ask interpreters not to let patients know that they have cancer, with some even threatening interpreters with consequences if they reveal the diagnosis. In such cases, the participants said that they would try to explain their role as interpreters in line with the Code of Ethics, as exemplified below:

> If I take Lebanon as an example, if one of your relatives has got, for example, cancer, you go to the doctor and talk to him at the side, please don't tell him because it will be so depressing to him, it might kill him. So, the doctor cooperates with you when it comes to that matter. Here, no. They know that it's straightforward. If there is some information to be informed to them, it has to be said. So, sometimes you find the relatives of that person telling me please don't tell the patient. But I tell them, I'm sorry, in my job I have to say everything that goes around here. It can't be a secret.
>
> (Participant 54, Arabic interpreter)

Moving on to the other strategy, 'interpreting everything as it is', data analysis indicates that this is considered synonymous with word-for-word interpreting among some interpreters. It can be best exemplified by feelings and emotions. In the case of Participant 6, a Korean interpreter, the interpreter reported '답답하다 (*dapdaphada*)' as untranslatable. The expression is commonly used by Korean people to express combined feelings of frustration, hopelessness, sadness and distress (Schmidt-Atzert & Park, 1999), yet the same expression can also be used to indicate feeling clogged up in the chest or feeling stuffy due to poor ventilation (Cho, 2024a). While there is not a single English expression that can accurately capture the multiple nuances of the word, its meaning is simplified and standardised in popular online translation apps. Google Translate, for example, recommends only one English expression, 'frustrated', for '답답하다'.

Even though the participant understood the inadequacy of the machine-translated expressions, the interpreter reported sticking to the word-for-word translation, citing that interpreters must deliver everything as it is. It can be conjectured that for English-speaking doctors who have no clue about the cultural complexity of certain words, the surface-level translations would 'make sense' for they are grammatically correct in English. The loss of cultural nuances in interpreting may, in turn, impact HCPs' understanding of the health conditions of NESB patients and may potentially influence diagnoses.

The machine-like strategy can also affect the comprehension of NESB patients particularly when it is used to translate unfamiliar medical concepts and terminologies. Mental illnesses, for example, are stigmatised in many societies and are treated as 'the unmentionable' (Cho, 2021). Furthermore, medical concepts of mental health in certain cultures significantly differ from the Australian context. Some commonly known conditions such as depression do not exist in many cultures and for many such societies, being mentally ill is synonymous with being 'crazy' (Mehraby, 2009).

Data analysis indicates that NESB patients from certain cultures have trouble understanding various concepts and names of mental illnesses as categorised in Australia. According to Participant 61, a Dari-Hazaragi interpreter, for example, people in Afghanistan are not familiar with commonly known conditions in Australia such as anxiety, depression and schizophrenia. While many of those terms have Afghan equivalents, they are used primarily among medical professionals and are not familiarised in the wider community. If these terms are interpreted as they are, many Afghan patients, therefore, would not understand them. When asked how he deals with communication problems in this respect, the interpreter said that he interprets as it is, leaving problems to be sorted out naturally through mutual clarification between the doctor and the patient:

> ... don't do anything. I use the actual word and I let, actually, the professional to explain it because that's how it works, and I interpret then the patient either gets confused or would ask me, sorry, I didn't understand it, then I have to get the professional to explain it and then I interpret the explanation.

While the strategy of 'interpreting as it is' is reported to work, it raises the question, what if patients do not seek clarification? It was, indeed, reported that NESB patients often do not ask doctors questions, even when they fail to understand. Reasons behind these reported observations include a lack of confidence, feeling inferior to doctors as the absolute authority, expectations of interpreters explaining everything, and not knowing their right to seek and receive clarification.

The possibility that patient responses to unclear messages vary is evident when comparing responses from the participants from the same country of origin. While the last-mentioned interpreter said that Afghan patients would ask for clarification, another (Participant 40) reported that many Afghan people do not seek clarifications for the reasons cited above. This indicates a possibility that some patients may miss out on important medical information, raising questions about the effectiveness of the strategy of 'interpreting as it is'. It may also compromise HCPs' abilities to accurately understand patient conditions due to the surface-level translations which, in turn, would potentially impact diagnoses and treatment of NESB patients.

6.3.2.2 Norm-adjusted strategies

The norm-adjusted strategies involve both independent strategies and collaborative strategies with HCPs (see Table 6.2). No norm-adjusted strategies are carried out with patients.

6.3.2.2.1 INDEPENDENT STRATEGIES

Under the category of independent strategies, there are two subcategories: self-contained versus open strategies. In self-contained strategies, the interpreter does not let other parties know the existence of the problems yet tries to handle communication problems on their own by approaching the Code flexibly. In open strategies, the interpreter remains flexible in their approaches by letting other parties know that there are communication problems. Other parties, i.e., HCPs, do not work together with interpreters to address communication problems. However, interpreters do necessary work to work out strategies, which distinguishes this strategy from 'collaborative strategies with HCPs'. Data analysis shows that self-contained strategies far outweigh open strategies (see Table 6.2). Whereas there are only two open strategies, there is a total of thirteen self-contained strategies. This raises the question of why the participants prefer to keep things to themselves rather than alerting other parties to the problems.

Data analysis indicates that the participants opt to work alone due to a lack of HCP willingness to learn about other cultures. It was reported that some HCPs do not welcome interpreters' suggestions regarding cultural differences and often cut short their explanations about cultural problems which affect communication. The lack of appreciation for culture among HCPs is exemplified by the following narrative:

> So, if you were to say, I'm sorry, you need to actually allow me to do the interpreting. You can't just – a few times you have said, I'm sorry, let me tell – and then they cut you off. They cut you off as though it's taking too long, yeah. They don't allow me to make them understand that there are some concepts that don't exist.
>
> (Participant 4, Farsi interpreter)

Working in the field in which established professionals hold more power, the participants reported that it is often easier to address problems on their own, rather than trying to involve HCPs who treat culture as irrelevant to interpreter-mediated communication. As for the specific strategies that they use in a self-contained manner, approximation is found to be useful to prompt HCPs to seek further clarification without letting them know the existence of the communication problem. This strategy is a modified version of the original intention of approximation, which refers to a strategy of trying to find a meaning close to the original meaning where full translation is tricky (As-Safi, 2011).

Taking Participant 32, an Indonesian interpreter, as an example, the interpreter reported approximating the meaning of *masuk angin*, literally meaning 'enter wind'. According to the participant, it refers to a combination of feeling chilly, heavy and sore all over the body, having gastric distress and experiencing headaches (see Wargadiredja, 2017). Known as an Indonesia-specific symptom, this condition is popularly believed to be caused by 'wind' or cold conditions (e.g., cold air, wet clothes, etc.) (Anggoro & Jee, 2021). While it includes some cold-like symptoms such as feeling chilly, it is distinguished from colds and flu among Indonesians (Anggoro & Jee, 2021). Pointing out *masuk angin* as a common challenge encountered by Indonesian interpreters, the participant warned against substituting the symptom as a cold, which she said some interpreters do, due to the complex meanings embedded in the term. The participant instead approximates it as 'under the weather', which often prompts HCPs to ask patients further questions to accurately understand the conditions. For example:

> I've heard some of my colleagues, other interpreters, they translate it as coming cold, but then when you say that, there is a possibility it's not even that. It's somewhat similar, but then the doctor would stop there and not ask further what they're actually having. To avoid that, I would usually say 'under the weather' and then the doctor gets to elaborate more. So I can maintain accuracy without actually leaving room for doctor to mistranslate what the patients say.

In certain cases, the participants reported mixing different strategies, rather than using a single one. Strategies are combined to deliver intended meanings most effectively. A case reported by Participant 23, a Turkish interpreter, offers a good example. According to the interpreter, doctors often ask patients 'if we lose you, would you like us to bring you back to life again through CPR?' as part of an informed consent process prior to major surgery. Pointing out that the expression might sound too confronting to elderly Turkish patients, the interpreter reported mixing the strategies of explaining meanings in detail and using lay terms through which to attenuate meanings. This way, the interpreter can deliver meanings without needing to explain cultural differences to HCPs as exemplified below:

> The CPR. If we lose you, would you like us to bring you back to life again? Bring you back to life, that's a bit harsh saying we want to bring you back to life. So instead of saying bring you back to life, I would say, if something happens to you and we feel that if you were to come back that you'd be really disabled or you'd be physically really disabled, would you like us to bring you back? I always say this is something that they say to a lot of their patients so that it's not just for them only. It's something that is disclosed to a lot of patients at his age or at his level of illness I suppose. Normally it's really elderly, anything over 80.

Some more inventive examples of self-contained strategies are found in strategies relating to gender and sex. In certain cultures, it is not appropriate for the opposite gender to mention or discuss issues relating to gender and sex (see Table 6.1). It was, however, reported that interpreters often have a client of the opposite gender for assignments and, in such cases, interpreters use various strategies.

First, when a specific body part is mentioned, the participants use props to point to the body part, rather than verbalising it. As Participant 46, a Tamil interpreter, reported, he uses anatomical models to show a female body part under discussion to avoid being culturally inappropriate. Second, euphemism is identified as a useful strategy particularly for telephone interpreting. As using props would not work for this type of interpreting, the participants use euphemistic expressions to avoid the risk of being culturally insensitive. As reported by Participant 11, a Rohingya interpreter, for example, the interpreter euphemises the female genital parts by using 'front passage' and 'back passage', which is commonly understood by the cultural group. Finally, nonverbal strategies such as a tone of voice and eye contact are identified as commonly used to deal specifically with sex-related issues. In the case of having patients who are sex workers, the participants reported that many patients feel ashamed and are hesitant to fully disclose their medical conditions caused by work. In such cases, some participants speak gently and softly to let patients know that "I don't judge you" in the expression of Participant 17, a Thai interpreter. If patients find it too embarrassing to discuss issues in detail, some interpreters use the strategy of avoiding eye contact, because looking directly into the eyes is too confronting in certain cultures.

Not all cultural challenges can, however, be addressed in a self-contained manner, and data analysis indicates that the participants resort to open strategies when participation by other parties is necessary to address the problems. As indicated above, there are two open strategies: i) offering cultural explanations to HCPs; ii) suggesting HCPs might like to hire another interpreter.

As for the first strategy of offering cultural explanations to HCPs, cultural beliefs in food having temperature are reported to require this strategy. The participants from Afghanistan, the Arab World, India, Indonesian and Iran collectively pointed out the common local belief that food has temperature, i.e., cold versus hot food. Taking Participant 34, a Hindi interpreter, as an example, the interpreter reported a cultural phenomenon in which people try to avoid food of a certain nature as a health risk. According to the interpreter, some fruits such as papayas and pineapples are categorised as hot food in India and are to be avoided by pregnant women due to the risk of miscarriage. As the cultural specificity is unfamiliar to many doctors in Australia, however, it often creates confusion for doctors and hinders communication. In such cases, the participants offer cultural explanations, yet without asking for permission from HCPs by speaking as a third person. For example:

> So that's also something that comes up from time to time. I say that to the professional and say look, this is the interpreter talking – I'm not interpreting – but we have in our culture that we say some food have a cold nature. Some food has a hot nature. So that's what she's referring to. Then I take myself out of the conversation so that the professional knows where the patient comes from.
>
> (Participant 7, Farsi interpreter)

As for the other strategy of asking HCPs to find another interpreter, this is used when interpreting is not feasible due to cultural differences. Taking Participant 44, a Cantonese interpreter, as an example, the interpreter reported a case in which a male client felt too embarrassed to discuss intimate sexual details during a consultation. As the communication stalled, the interpreter decided to withdraw and suggested that the doctor hire another interpreter. This represents a slight modification of the Code of Conduct, which allows the interpreter to withdraw in case the interpreter's neutrality is compromised, or the interpreter's professional competence is not sufficient to manage a given assignment.

Data analysis indicates that the participants came up with various independent strategies by necessity to balance the competing needs of individual *illusio*, professional *illusio* and HCP expectations. By using these strategies, the participants feel they can achieve the goal of helping NESB migrants without compromising professional norms too much, while also satisfying HCP expectations of interpreting.

6.3.2.2.2 COLLABORATIVE STRATEGIES WITH HCPS

While many participants are found to work independently, a group of interpreters reported working together with HCPs to address cultural problems. Data analysis indicates a total of three strategies: i) asking HCPs to simplify terms; ii) pre-discussion with HCPs about tricky cultural issues; and iii) explaining to HCPs why patients are having trouble understanding the interpreting to find the optimal ways to address problems collaboratively.

As for the first strategy, asking HCPs to simplify terms, the participants reported using this strategy if medical terminology unfamiliar to patients was being used by HCPs. As verbatim interpreting would not make sense to patients, the participants said that they ask HCPs to use lay terms by explaining cultural unfamiliarity associated with them. This is exemplified by the case of Participant 30, an Arabic interpreter. According to the interpreter, 'lupus' is not commonly known in many Arabic-speaking countries and delivering the medically defined equivalent of the term is highly unlikely to be understood by patients. As such, the rationale behind the strategy is to make information more accessible to NESB patients.

The second strategy of having pre-discussions with HCPs about certain cultural issues is found to be useful to avoid misunderstandings by patients and for its positive impact on communication. Cancer was reported as the most frequent source of communication problems. The participants reported that they discussed potential problems with HCPs before interpreting to ensure their cultural appropriateness. The strategy was reported to be used only if HCPs appear to be aware of the cultural significance of cancer. For example:

> If the doctor is culturally aware of the sensitivities towards the illness, cancer, in terms of the Greek understanding, a lot of times I have to take the doctor on the side and say have you had a chat with the family? Is it okay for me to address this issue? There are times that the patient can even pass away without knowing what he or she has been suffering from. It's the unspoken word I would say.
>
> (Participant 25, Greek interpreter)

Finally, it was reported that patients with a low level of education often find it difficult to follow medical communication. In such cases, the participants point out the underlying issue to HCPs to collaboratively find ways to make communication work for NESB patients. According to the participants, many migrants, particularly elderly migrants, do not have much education and have trouble understanding complex words even in their own language. When the problem is apparent to interpreters, they step in to alert HCPs to a patient's limited capacity to understand communication as exemplified below:

> It's extremely important that they [interpreters] deliver the message the way it is without changing it or you know, possibly even better if you can translate exact words of the health care provider. Then maybe if the patient says sorry, I don't understand what you're saying. Take a minute and explain [to] the doctor he doesn't understand because he's confused or he doesn't have the vocabulary, he doesn't have the education, you know? But I also think that a lot of interpreters at the beginning are very much afraid of taking this time because they could see that their role is absolutely to translate literally what the health care providers or the lawyers say and stick to it, otherwise you will not be professional. And I think that you can be very professional and also do this, I mean even more professional because if you're translating something and you know that the person is not understanding what you're saying, where is the professionality? What is the point?
>
> (Participant 39, Italian interpreter)

The strategies are found to be geared towards helping NESB patients, indicating the personal-level *illusio* as a key motivation behind the interpreting decisions. These strategies also serve as a good example of managing culture-related communication through inter-party collaboration between interpreters and HCPs.

6.3.2.3 Norm-resistant strategies

Under this category, there are three types of strategies: i) sharing interpreters' own experiences with patients; ii) making suggestions to HCPs to modify test items to suit the cultural needs of patients; and iii) exercising extra care for patients outside consultations. While the first and third strategies are found to be independently carried out by interpreters, the second strategy is collaborative by involving HCPs.

According to the Code, the principle of role boundaries mandates interpreters to maintain clear boundaries as a communication facilitator without getting involved in other tasks unrelated to interpreting (see

Australian Institute of Interpreters and Translators, 2012). The Code also emphasises that in any work arrangement which goes against this tenet, practitioners are required to explain their role boundaries by drawing a clear demarcation between interpreting and other tasks. In this regard, any of the identified strategies might constitute a breach of the Code. It is, however, important to ask why the participants are willing to step out of their role as an interpreter, and this section examines this very question.

To begin with, the strategy in which interpreters share their personal experiences with patients was reported to be useful to deal with elderly migrants who have a culturally ingrained fear of nursing homes. While moving to aged care facilities later in life is generally considered a regular step in Australia, nursing homes are culturally feared in many societies as a place for people with no hope of life (Cho, 2024b). Due to such negative cultural associations, it was reported that many elderly migrants try to avoid having anything to do with nursing homes, and this creates challenges in the case of cognitive assessments of elderly patients.

According to the participants, elderly clients are often reluctant to cooperate with assessment processes, fearing that test results might impact their wish to stay at home and lead to being forced into nursing homes. As a result, many patients are not fully transparent about how they manage daily tasks. In some cases, elderly clients even refuse to take tests, fearing that any association with assessments would increase their chances of being sent to nursing homes. It was reported that if elderly people are informed of what assessments are about, i.e., not designed to send people to nursing homes, many are willing and cooperative. Some participants, therefore, try to help patients understand cultural differences relating to nursing homes between the home country and the host society. They reported using personal approaches such as sharing their own experiences relating to Australian aged care facilities to address patients' fears. For example:

> It involves a lot of care talking, you can soften your language, you try to break the friendliness barrier or whatever, just trying to get into their confidence in order to pass the message on [...] Therefore, it's probably helpful as well to explain that. From the experiences that I have had myself with my own family, my own father who is at the respite end of the nursing home and so forth, that is something that I see that they really appreciate, or that it's much easier for me to explain how this place looks, what this place does, where they are, how the members of family can visit, they can take them out for the day if they want to and how they will exist if they ever need to go into this facility.
>
> (Participant 57, Polish interpreter)

Moving on to the second strategy, suggesting HCPs modify test items, the participants reported that some items of cognitive assessments for elderly people are not culturally informed, putting NESB elderly patients at a disadvantage. It was reported that certain cultural items such as Australian food (e.g., Vegemite) are not familiar to older migrants who stick to their original lifestyles (see also Cho, 2024a). If elderly people are given the task of recalling food items for a memory test, for example, the lack of cultural familiarity was said to affect their test performances. In the case of Participant 39, an Italian interpreter, the interpreter noticed that 'tea' was often used for a memory assessment test in Australia. As coffee is a lot more common in Italy, the interpreter discussed the problem with HCPs prior to a test to avoid potential disadvantages for elderly patients. Similarly, Participant 53, a Polish interpreter, reported that he usually suggests replacing unfamiliar Australian food items with a familiar food such as a *pierogi*, a Polish dumpling.

As for the final strategy, that of showing extra care outside consultations, it was reported that many migrant patients are not familiar with common types of medicine in Australia. Furthermore, NESB patients' lack of proficiency in English makes it difficult for them to remember names of medicine discussed during consultations. It is particularly problematic for purchasing over-the-counter medicine, which does not require prescriptions bearing the names of medicine. As most medicine has complex English names, it is not easy for NESB patients to recall them. To help such patients, some interpreters such as Participant 37, a Thai interpreter, offer to write down the names of medicine for patients after the consultation. She also tries to teach patients how to pronounce the names of medicine by phonetically writing them down in Thai.

Relatedly, some interpreters reported sharing free medical services relevant to patients' conditions after consultations. The participants pointed to a lack of general knowledge about the Australian health care system among migrant patients as a significant problem which affects NESB patient access to health information. It was reported that common expressions such as GP (General Practitioner) are not familiar to many people, and consultations with NESB patients with inadequate knowledge about Australian medical systems, therefore, require more time than regular consultations. As doctors tend to run behind schedule, however, NESB patients are often unable to find opportunities to discuss their health concerns fully (see Section 5.4). The allocation of the standard consultation time of 15 minutes to interpreter-assisted consultations also contributes to the lack of time for patients to fully discuss their health concerns (see Section 5.4). In the case of Participant 56, a Cambodian interpreter, the interpreter recalled the case of a patient with sexual health issues. The interpreter said that the patient seemed very worried after the consultation because she did not have enough time to discuss her concerns. Feeling sorry for the patient, the interpreter advised the patient to go to a government-run sexual health clinic which provides free information on sexual health, knowing that his action constitutes 'breach of the Code':

> Yes, I do understand that I sometimes breach the codes as well because then I sort of you know what? We do have also a sexual health clinic that can also provide free information about this as well. This is all that I can say. I wouldn't recommend ... any clinic but just saying to them that the government here, we do also have a sexual health clinic. We can provide a health information in regard to your diagnosis. Do you want me to ask that question to the front desk and the front desk can direct you to the right clinic? Most of the time, client will say yes, yes. Please ask them that and then I explain that to the front desk. Front desk will then give them the phone number for them to get in touch and so on. So that sort of a mini light bulb that I lit for client that hey, I won't help you but sort of that's a different way to help them out.

Data analysis indicates that the norm-resistant strategies are the outcome of the personal-level *illusio* of helping others. As exemplified above, the expressed beliefs in the worthiness of looking after NESB patients are in line with the identified *illusio* relating to helping migrants, highlighting the strong workings of personal-level *illusio* on interpreters' decisions. It also shows that the communication needs of NESB patients are not limited to consultation settings and may extend beyond scheduled meetings. As there are hardly any guidelines on these specific needs, the participants decided to take actions in line with their personal commitment to the field.

Overall, data analysis indicates incompatibility between personal commitment, professional norms and institutional monolingualism. These conflicts are seen to lead many interpreters to come up with their own strategies to deal with communication problems in their own ways. It indicates interpreting as solo work, as exemplified by the disproportionately high number of independent strategies. This raises the question of how to promote inter-party collaboration between interpreters and HCPs, and the next section aims to answer it.

6.4 Ways to work together

Data analysis indicates that the participants generally think that the inter-party collaboration is a good idea, yet they pointed out the institutional lack of appreciation for and understanding about interpreting as a formidable obstacle. To achieve this goal, many participants highlighted the importance of training HCPs in interpreting. It was reported that health care interpreters in Australia are required to learn about how to work with HCPs and need to regularly update their medical knowledge as part of their professional recertification requirements. It was, however, pointed out that HCPs are generally not required to be trained in how to work with interpreters. According to Participant 10, a Spanish interpreter who has done research on interpreter engagement in Australian health care as part of her previous government job, training opportunities regarding interpreting for HCPs are rare and, even if they are available, many HCPs are not keen to learn about interpreting.

When it comes to how to train HCPs, the participants made the following five recommendations: increase cultural awareness; understand the importance of an optimal environment for interpreting; speak at the level of patients; understand interpreting challenges; and finally, recognise interpreting as a legitimate profession.

First, increasing cultural awareness was said to be important, particularly for problems which have a significant cultural gap such as delivering a bad diagnosis (e.g., cancer). Many participants expressed the emotional toll that it often takes to break bad news to patients who are not used to the Australian norm. While many believed that it is important for patients to know the truth, breaking news too abruptly without considering the patient's culture was reported as an area of consideration to improve health care for migrant patients. To this end, the participants suggested holding regular forums to provide HCPs with cultural knowledge based on interpreters' professional experiences. For example:

> It's absolutely necessary for them to understand. So, for me having a forum of different interpreters from different languages to come up with examples, have a panel and have quite a few of these sessions for them that you could bring three or four different languages each time for them to make them understand, because the problems that I would have in Persian are not the problems that somebody in Bengali would have.
>
> (Participant 4, Farsi interpreter)

Second, it was recommended that the current work environment for interpreters be enhanced to make it more conducive for interpreters to perform their work to the best of their abilities. Many pointed out the need for briefing, which was said to exist only in the guidelines and hardly ever provided to interpreters. Furthermore, HCPs were urged to secure a quiet environment and ensure good sound quality, especially for telephone interpreting work. This relates to the need for HCPs to understand the importance of communication for health care, particularly the specific needs of interpreter-mediated communication settings. For example:

> For me one of the main things is that they need to understand that it's all about communication. If you want the interpreter to facilitate communication, you have to make sure that the interpreter can in fact communicate first of all. If you are using a telephone where you can hardly hear, that's not good for interpreting. The interpreter will need to hear better than in a normal situation because you need to process the information, reformulate it.
>
> (Participant 2, Spanish interpreter)

Third, it was suggested that HCPs make communication more interpreter-friendly and, importantly, more patient-friendly. The participants pointed out the general tendency among HCPs to overuse complex medical terminologies and concepts. Whilst acknowledging the importance of acquiring and updating medical knowledge, many participants said that it would be impractical to expect interpreters to be as knowledgeable as HCPs about medical practice. Even if interpreters manage to deliver complex terminology in the language of patients, it was reported that many patients have trouble understanding due to cultural unfamiliarity and a low level of education. Problematising the common perception of interpreters as translation machines, the participants stressed that simpler languages would make it easy for both interpreters and patients, as exemplified below:

> I think they think if you are an interpreter, you know everything. We are human beings too. They can't expect us to have that much knowledge, being an interpreter. I think maybe to be mindful that interpreters won't know each and every thing and they need to explain them.
>
> (Participant 45, Tamil interpreter)

Another area of improvement to facilitate inter-party collaboration is to enhance HCPs' understandings about the challenges of interpreting. It was reported that the dominant tendency to view interpreters as translation machines leads to the perception among HCPs that interpreting is automatic and must be error-free. Challenges resulting from working with HCPs who knew little about interpreting, not to mention its challenges, were found to be all too common. According to the participants, the dominant view of interpreters as machines and communication as the interpreter's responsibilities are deeply entrenched in the current milieu of Australian health care. Under such circumstances, any communication problems tend to be seen as interpreter faults, as exemplified below:

> We, as interpreters, we are the meat in the middle of the sandwich. We are the only people that are always being blamed for not doing the job properly.
>
> (Participant 3, Farsi interpreter)

Finally, it was emphasised that HCPs need to recognise interpreters as full-fledged professionals. Concerns were expressed about the way in which interpreters are treated as something other than what they really are. As amply demonstrated throughout this book, interpreters are seen as machines, some sort of bilingual, or as semi-professionals. Furthermore, interpreting is often seen as unnecessary by HCPs, a time waster and an inconvenience. Critical of the current institutional perception and treatment of interpreting and interpreters, the participants emphasised the need for interpreting to be properly recognised by enhancing HCPs' awareness of interpreting:

> I think just to make them aware a situation [that does occur] from time to time. We need to give them extra time, and we need to acknowledge and welcome that other person in the room that is helping their client.
>
> (Participant 57, Polish interpreter)

It is important to note a striking similarity between these recommendations from the participants and those from the first health care interpreters in the 1970s (see Section 3.3). Similar to the recommendations from the interpreters today, the early health care interpreters emphasised the importance of training for HCPs. The earlier suggestions include:

- Training of health care professionals regarding cultural sensitivity of NESB patients
- Awareness-raising among health care professionals regarding the importance of interpreting
- Improvement of publicity and public education regarding the necessity for interpreting services
- More engagement of interpreters in health care interactions as co-professionals
- Removal of racial biases against interpreters and interpreting services as special schemes for migrants
- An increase in the number of health care interpreters
- Training for interpreters regarding medical expertise and interaction handling

As can be seen above, many of the suggestions from the contemporary interpreters had previously been proposed, with the emphasis placed on the need to train HCPs in culture, better awareness of interpreting and professional legitimacy. It suggests that while Australia has achieved a lot in terms of establishing the interpreting system, little has changed in terms of the institutional awareness of and practice with interpreting.

In an environment in which interpreting is understood so little, most interpreters work alone, rather than working together, as exemplified by the findings from this chapter. The normalisation of interpreting as solo work may, in turn, further contribute to institutional disinterest and the resultant under-recognition of interpreting. Training of HCPs is, therefore, urgently needed:

> So, I guess, training, and training for these health care professionals, be it doctors, be it nurses, they're the ones that need more understanding. I mean, these are the patients of the facility, and whether they speak the language, or not speak the language, they need to receive the same treatment. We are all on the same page like that. Better understanding, and better culturally appropriate health care setting, is what we do need.
>
> (Participant 48, Tagalog interpreter)

As accentuated in this narrative, everyone needs to be treated equally, particularly in health care, to ensure individuals have the ability to lead the life they deserve as human beings. Disregarding interpreting and the specific needs of interpreters have direct implications for the quality of care which NESB patients receive. The under-appreciation of interpreting is, indeed, equated with the under-recognition of the rights of marginalised populations, and the chapter highlights the urgent need to bring about changes to the institutional perception and treatment of interpreting in Australian health care.

6.5 Summary

The chapter investigated how individually held meanings of interpreting intersect with professional norms and institutional monolingualism and how their interactions influence the ways interpreters work. Conflicts are found to often arise when interpreters navigate communication problems relating to culture, leading interpreters to invent various strategies to bridge the gap between the personal, the professional and the institutional. The chapter has made four important discoveries.

First, the personal-level *illusio* illuminates why many interpreters stay committed to the field, namely to help vulnerable populations, despite the general under-recognition of the profession. Data analysis indicates that interpreters who are linguistically, ethnically and culturally aligned with NESB migrants are committed to helping the marginalised by utilising their bilingual skills. As amply illustrated, many participants who came to Australia as migrants not proficient in English were deeply sympathetic with the struggles of NESB populations and saw interpreting as their moral obligation to help their ethnic communities. The findings show the important roles that interpreting plays in promoting ethnic empowerment and access equity in English-monolingual Australia, where communication problems and other struggles of NESB migrants remain under-acknowledged.

Second, analysis of the interactions between personal aspirations, professional norms and institutional monolingualism indicates conflicts between those three elements. Such incompatibility is found to have pushed interpreters to come up with their own strategies to handle communication problems. Analysis indicates a lack of balance between the identified strategies, with most falling into the category of independent, norm-adjusted strategies. Interpreters are found to work mostly on their own to adjust the professional norms without involving those HCPs who fail to see the importance of culture to communication. This confirms interpreting as solo work, and this is, indeed, in line with the institutional expectation of interpreting.

The findings also indicate inverted relations specifically between the personal-level *illusio* and the professional norm. That is, the strategies which are closest to the norm, i.e., norm-oriented strategies, are found to be least influenced by the personal *illusio*, whereas the strategies which are furthest away from the norm, norm-resistant strategies, are in line with the personal aspiration of helping NESB patients. While it is not the intention of this chapter to judge which strategies are better, it is important to pay attention to the potential impact of the norm-oriented strategies on communication. Taking machine-like interpreting as an example, while the strategy might technically be in line with the accuracy norm, it risks misrepresenting patients' health conditions due to the oversimplification or distortion of meanings that often result from word-for-word interpreting. It is also important to note a lack of specific guidelines on how to address NESB patients' communication needs, which go beyond consultation settings. The current Code of Ethics focuses exclusively on interpreter-mediated communication settings, and the findings indicate the need to extend the boundary of communication for NESB patients by considering their specific needs.

A third discovery highlighted by analysis of the data is the need to improve HCP awareness of interpreter-mediated communications including the importance of culture and knowledge about interpreting. As a space where different languages and cultures constantly interact, interpreting inevitably encounters communication problems arising from these interactions. As amply illustrated, culture is, however, generally seen by HCPs to be irrelevant to communication, which, in turn, impacts interpreters' abilities to handle sensitive cultural problems appropriately. The identified lack of cultural awareness among HCPs in this chapter is in line with the findings from Chapter 5 in which interpreting is predominantly seen as a word-for-word exercise and interpreters as translation machines. It is, therefore, important to improve cultural awareness among HCPs by considering specific communication issues which arise in interpreting.

Relatedly and finally, the chapter highlights the importance of training HCPs in interpreting and working with interpreters. The identified lack of knowledge about interpreting among HCPs is concerning, considering the long history of health care interpreting in Australia. As the world's first provision of language services for migrants, health care interpreting has consistently developed throughout the past five decades, as exemplified by the establishment of various governing, certification and professional systems (see Sections 3.2 and 3.4). As demonstrated in this chapter, however, the systemic development of health care interpreting services has not been matched by the corresponding awareness of people with whom interpreters work. The gap is all the more important when considering the high level of resemblance between the recommendations made by the participants in this study and those from the first health care interpreting services in the 1970s (see Section 3.3).

Considering this striking resemblance, it is entirely possible that not much has been done in terms of promoting HCPs' awareness of interpreting. This emphasises interpreting as one significantly neglected area in Australian health care, calling for the need to bridge the gap by developing and mandating interpreting-related training for HCPs.

References

Anggoro, F. K., & Jee, B. D. (2021). The substance of cold: Indonesians' use of cold weather theory to explain everyday illnesses. *Frontiers in Psychology*, *12*, 734044. https://doi.org/10.3389/fpsyg.2021.734044

As-Safi, A. B. (2011). *Translation theories: Strategies and basic theoretical issues*. Al Manhal.

Australian Institute of Interpreters and Translators. (2012). *AUSIT Code of Ethics and Code of Conduct*. https://ausit.org/wp-content/uploads/2024/09/AUSIT-Code-of-Ethics-and-Code-of-Conduct.pdf

Bourdieu, P. (1998). *Practical reason: On the theory of action*. Polity Press.

Bourdieu, P. (2000). *Pascalian meditations*. Polity Press.

Bourdieu, P., & Wacquant, L. J. D. (1992). *An invitation to reflexive sociology*. Polity Press.

Cameron, M. E., & Namdul, T. (n.d.). *Tibetan Medicine*. www.takingcharge.csh.umn.edu/what-do-i-need-know-about-my-unique-constitution#:~:text=The%20five%20elements%20of%20earth,that%20are%20essential%20for%20life

Cho, J. (2021). *Intercultural communication in interpreting: Power and choices*. Routledge. https://doi.org/10.4324/9781003179993

Cho, J. (2023). Interpreters as translation machines: Telephone interpreting challenges as awareness problems. *Qualitative Health Research*, *33*(12), 1037–1048. https://doi.org/10.1177/10497323231191712

Cho, J. (2024a). Healthcare interpreting for Korean immigrants in Australia: Linguistic and cultural perspectives. In R. Moratto, & H.-O. Lim (Eds.), *The Routledge handbook of Korean interpreting* (pp. 245–257). Routledge. https://doi.org/10.4324/9781003349723-20

Cho, J. (2024b). To act or not to act: Interpreters' dilemmas and choices in aged care assessments of elderly migrants. *Journal of Multilingual and Multicultural Development*, *45*(7), 2412–2426. https://doi.org/10.1080/01434632.2022.2050916

Colley, H. (2012). Not learning in the workplace: Austerity and the shattering of illusio in public service work. *Journal of Workplace Learning*, *24*, 317–337. https://doi.org/10.1108/13665621211239868

Colley, H., & Guéry, F. (2015). Understanding new hybrid professions: Bourdieu, illusio and the case of public service interpreters. *Cambridge Journal of Education*, *45*(1), 113–131. https://doi.org/10.1080/0305764X.2014.991277

Connolly, D. J., Allen-Collinson, J., & Evans, A. B. (2016). A level playing 'field'? A Bourdieusian analysis of the career aspirations of further education students on sports courses. *Sport, Education and Society*, *21*(8), 1144–1160. https://doi.org/10.1080/13573322.2014.994175

Lupu, I., & Empson, L. (2015). Illusio and overwork: Playing the game in the accounting field. *Accounting, Auditing & Accountability Journal*, *28*(8), 1310–1340. https://doi.org/10.1108/AAAJ-02-2015-1984

Mehraby, N. (2009). Possessed or crazy? Mental illness across cultures. *Psychotherapy in Australia*, *15*(2), 43.

Nölleke, D., Maares, P., & Hanusch, F. (2022). Illusio and disillusionment: Expectations met or disappointed among young journalists. *Journalism*, *23*(2), 320–336. https://doi.org/10.1177/1464884920956820

Schmidt-Atzert, L., & Park, H. S. (1999). The Korean concepts dapdaphada and uulhada: A cross-cultural study of the meaning of emotions. *Journal of Cross-Cultural Psychology*, *30*(5), 646–654. https://doi.org/10.1177/0022022199030005006

Ulaş, A. P., & Gündüz, A. (2020). A bourdieusian perspective on the public service interpreters working at the non-governmental organizations. *Çeviribilim ve Uygulamaları Dergisi*, *28*, 144–176. https://doi.org/10.37599/ceviri.675408

Wargadiredja, A. T. (2017). *We Asked an Expert to Explain, Medically, What Happens When You Catch Masuk Angin.* www.vice.com/en/article/we-asked-an-expert-to-explain-medically-what-happens-when-you-catch-masuk-angin/

7 Multilingual understanding of monolingualism

7.1 Interpreting monolingualism

In Chapter 1, I asked the following key questions. First, why is interpreting under-appreciated in Australia despite its centrality to the social inclusion of migrants? Second, how does the under-recognition of interpreting impact the ways interpreters work? Third, how does the under-recognition of interpreting relate to broader social attitudes to other languages and speakers in Australia? The critical sociolinguistic examination of these questions shows that the under-appreciation of interpreting relates profoundly to the monolingualism which is embedded in linguistic, racial and class hierarchies in Australian society. The investigation of the under-recognition of interpreting in various social and professional spaces of interpreting emphasises interpreting as a space of inequalities which disproportionately impact migrants, including the interpreters themselves.

Monolingualism in each space carries distinctive ideological features and has different impacts on interpreting and interpreters. Importantly, these ideologies are inter-linked across all spaces, highlighting the insidious nature and pervasiveness of monolingualism in Australian society. The distinctive dimensions of monolingualism and its clearly identified ties with interpreting are set out in the following four sub-sections.

7.1.1 Societal monolingualism

Monolingualism is commonly associated with language, but this book demonstrates that monolingualism is not just about language but strongly relates to racial and class biases against migrants. By examining the processes by which English has intersected with racial and class hierarchies within the migration history of Australia, Chapter 3 highlights how English monolingualism is an outcome of Australia's pursuit of social homogeneity characterised by British identity and whiteness. In the process of building a white nation (Hage, 2012), English was entrenched as

DOI: 10.4324/9781032614854-7

a key tool to maintain and strengthen the homogeneity of the evolving society. English was used to keep out the undesirable, while simultaneously imposing itself on NESB migrants in the nation to promote social homogeneity through linguistic unity. Throughout these processes, English became racialised as a white language and served as a class maker, which distinguished Australians from ignorant migrants unable to speak English.

The naturalisation of linguistic, racial and class hierarchies in English is attributable to the unique sociohistorical conditions of Australia primarily characterised by the 'White Australia' policy. Representing an unprecedented social engineering project in modern history, White Australia is found to provide a fertile ground for English monolingualism to be entrenched and strengthened. NESB migrants struggled enormously, yet migrants were blamed for failing to assimilate and were generally regarded as social problems under White Australia. The lack of understanding of language barriers and migrant struggles impacted the development of interpreting too. Within the monolingual societal milieu, the need for formal language service provision was ignored, and it was not until communication issues became too serious to be denied that the government finally decided to begin language services for migrants.

The formalisation of the health care interpreting services in 1977 signified a new era in which diversity was officially embraced in multicultural Australia (Clyne, 1991). As part of the earlier multicultural policy initiatives, significant progress was achieved in terms of policy and systemic development relating to interpreting. Such progress, however, failed to translate into corresponding public awareness about linguistic diversity, language barriers and interpreting. The long-standing ignorance and suppression of other languages and speakers were too deeply entrenched and continued to be strengthened in 'multicultural Australia' in which the proportion of migrants significantly increased. Without concerted government-level efforts to promote public awareness of diversity and inclusion, the social biases infiltrated into various domains of Australian society and the book identifies health care as one key carrier of societal monolingualism.

Australian health care had long been English-monolingual and Anglocentric by the time health care interpreting was introduced. As a result, the emerging profession of interpreting suffered from the linguistic, class and racial biases already entrenched within the health care system. The examination of the experiences of the first health care interpreters in the 1970s shows that these interpreters were subject to various biases, which identified them as aligned with uneducated migrants. Due to the generally migrant profile of interpreters and the migrants they served, interpreting was regarded as a temporary welfare scheme for poor migrants who could not speak English, rather than a genuine profession. Apart from the racial and class biases against interpreting, a significant lack of awareness and understanding of other languages and speakers within Australian hospitals also contributed to the challenges encountered by the early interpreters. Interpreters were not treated as professional equals by health care practitioners who saw them as threats to their exclusive power, time wasters and necessary evils. The book illuminates how interpreting became racialised and hierarchised professionally within the traditionally English-monolingual environment of Australian health care.

The poor perception of interpreting persists into the current era. While the interpreting provision system has achieved internal progress over the past five decades, as exemplified by the establishment of various professional and governing bodies, external awareness and recognition of interpreting remain problematic. Interpreting continues to be treated as a semi-profession, with the lack of professional legitimacy representing a significant source of frustration for interpreters in Australia (Eser & Lai, 2018; Hale & Napier, 2016; Rodriguez-Losada, 2019).

The exposure of the ties between societal monolingualism and interpreting indicates the under-appreciation of interpreting in Australian society as a sociolinguistic problem relating to entrenched biases against other languages and speakers. It shows that ongoing under-recognition of interpreting is deeply rooted in the sociohistorical and sociolinguistic conditions of Australia, confirming that the under-appreciation of interpreting is a manifestation of monolingual biases, which are both historical and contemporary.

7.1.2 Market monolingualism

Having identified the impacts of societal monolingualism on interpreting, the book moved on in Chapter 4 to explore market monolingualism in the Australian interpreting market. The examination of the material conditions of interpreting in the market found that interpreting and related bilingual skills are profoundly under-recognised. Interpreting is generally seen as a job that any bilingual person can manage and bilingualism tends to be treated as a non-skill. While it takes a lot of investment and hard work to become an interpreter in Australia, the market does not generally require interpreting certifications for interpreter recruitment. This has, in turn, allowed non-professionals who claim to be bilingual to enter the market, leading to market disruption and disorganisation.

The book shows that the lack of regard for interpreting and bilingual skills is strongly to do with racial and class biases against migrant workers. The shift in seeing interpreters from language professionals to bilingual migrant workers illuminates the racialised and class-based workings of market monolingualism, which treats interpreters as migrant workers and, as a consequence, significantly under-appreciates them. This is most evident in the low rate of pay for interpreting, which is not commensurate with the generally high level of education that the participants have received. While the deterioration in the interpreting rate and working conditions is attributable to the neoliberal restructuring of the Australian interpreting sector (see Section 3.4), the mismatch between the market reality and the professional and educational qualifications of interpreters is a key signifier of market practice as discriminatory against migrants. The constant flow of bilingual migrants in search of jobs also only serves to strengthen the market's practices. As extensively illustrated, it is difficult for migrants to find decent work in Australia and many end up entering the interpreting market as an interim pathway until they find a better job. Gender is identified as another factor which leads migrant women to pursue interpreting due to the flexibility of the profession. As these job-seeking migrants represent a reliable source of supply, the market has little motivation to change its current practice, reinforcing the view of interpreting and language as a non-skill.

Chapter 4 also shows that market monolingualism is strongly tied to societal monolingualism. As amply exemplified in Chapter 3, the long-standing biases against other languages and their speakers in Australian society have rendered interpreting invisible and irrelevant to mainstream life. Furthermore, the traditional association of interpreting with migrants is found to reinforce public disinterest in interpreting in Australia. The racial and class-based workings of societal monolingualism are found to be replicated within the interpreting market, which subjects bilingual migrant workers to linguistic, racial and class biases. The concentration of migrants in the interpreting market is shown to strengthen and reinforce market monolingualism and the consequential under-valuation of interpreting.

The generally low status of interpreting has been attributed to various systemic aspects of interpreting (Dam, 2017; D'Hayer, 2012; Hlavac, 2015; Mikkelson, 1996), yet the book proves that market monolingualism is one of the most significant factor behind the under-appreciation of interpreting. By examining the ties between interpreting and migration within the interpreting market, the chapter defines market monolingualism as a racialised and class-based practice. While non-professional interpreters tend to be blamed as obstacles to the development of interpreting as a fully fledged profession, the focus on the migrant aspects of interpreting shows that it is not necessarily uncertified interpreters but market monolingualism which is singled out as a significant obstacle to the development of interpreting as a legitimate profession.

7.1.3 Institutional monolingualism

Moving on to Australian health care institutions, the book highlights a significant lack of knowledge about interpreting in Australian hospitals. Chapter 5 shows that at all levels of Australian hospitals, interpreting is not properly understood and frequently overlooked. The old practice of using any bilinguals as interpreters is found to continue among HCPs, especially front desk staff and doctors. Training for HCPs in the use and value of interpreting is recommended by relevant health guidelines, yet the findings indicate that many doctors do not understand the very basic needs of interpreters such as the need to hear clearly to interpret properly. Rather than viewed as human language professionals, interpreters are typically regarded as translation machines, with interpreting seen as automated activities unaffected by unfavourable external conditions.

The identified lack of respect for interpreting and interpreters is a case of *déjà vu*. Health care interpreters in the past, as illustrated in Chapter 3, suffered from a lack of professional legitimacy and inadequate understanding of the role among HCPs. Fifty years on, interpreters working within contemporary Australian hospitals are found to experience the same problems. Australia is regarded as a global leader in terms of language provision services, yet the book highlights a significant gap between the system, which is regarded as a model, and the actual level of awareness and treatment of interpreting within health care institutions.

The effects of institutional monolingualism within Australian hospitals are further demonstrated by the racial and class-based workings of English monolingualism against NESB patients. Patients not fluent in English are found to be subject to monolingual biases, even in the presence of interpreters. The identified lack of respect for patients not proficient in English among front desk staff and doctors is reminiscent of the past practice in which NESB patients were treated as a "'second class citizenship'" (Hearn, 1981, p. 7, emphasis in original).

The impact of institutional monolingualism on minority patients in interpreter-mediated communications is further highlighted by systemic problems in Australian health care. Interpreter-mediated consultations need to be prioritised to allow interpreters to finish a given assignment on time so that interpreters can leave for the next assignment as scheduled. This basic need in interpreter's work is, however, found to be unmet, forcing interpreters to wait for a long time for a consultation and to leave an assignment before it is finished. This will subsequently impact NESB patients who are unable to express themselves without interpreters. Furthermore, hospitals allocate the standard duration of fifteen minutes to interpreter-assisted consultations, rather than longer consultations. As interpreters need to repeat what was said, parties have only half the allotted time for communication, depriving NESB patients of opportunities to receive proper health care.

Migrants who are not fluent in the language of the host society tend to be subject to discrimination, yet their social experiences often remain unheard due to their inability to express themselves. The discovery of inequalities experienced by NESB patients in Australian health care through the eyes of interpreters is, therefore, extremely valuable, highlighting the relevance and importance of critical sociolinguistic approaches to interpreting.

It has been fifty years since the health care interpreter services began in Australia, and this book demonstrates that little progress has been achieved in terms of institutional perception and awareness of interpreting. Australian health care remains a fundamentally monolingual environment where the historical patterns of perceiving and treating other languages and speakers as irrelevant continue. These discoveries both represent how and explain why interpreting remains under-appreciated in Australia. The chapter highlights interpreting problems not just as occupational problems but as problems of access inequity and social justice for vulnerable populations.

7.1.4 Individual responses to monolingualism

Following the examination of monolingualism in various social and professional spaces of interpreting, the book explores how interpreters respond to monolingualism, specifically within the market and hospitals. To begin with, interpreters' responses to market monolingualism in Chapter 4 reveal that interpreters try to reconcile with the market reality owing to their own migrant status. While most participants were critical of the under-appreciation of interpreting within the market, the inherently disparate nature of the multi-ethnic and freelancing employment of interpreting makes it difficult for interpreters to accumulate significant power to force the market to change. Under such circumstances, interpreters try to compromise in relation to their given circumstances. The compromises are financial, gendered or community-giving, all of which relate to the migrant status of the interpreters themselves. Once again, the strong ties between migration and interpreting help sustain and reinforce market monolingualism.

Second, interpreter responses to the institutional monolingualism analysed in Chapter 6 highlight the gap between personal commitment and professional norms, one which tends to widen within the monolingual milieu of Australian health care. Asking why interpreters stay in the profession despite its general under-appreciation reveals the humanistic dimension of helping NESB migrants as the most significant factor behind interpreters' commitment to the field. Once again, the ties between interpreting and migration strongly figure in the examination. The participants, who formerly experienced struggles as new arrivals in Australia, are found to be sympathetic with the struggles of migrants from their ethnic community and to see interpreting as a key tool to enable access equity for vulnerable populations. This personal aspiration is, however, found to conflict with professional norms. Furthermore, institutional monolingualism characterised by inadequate awareness of cultural and linguistic diversity poses a significant obstacle to interpreters' work.

Such conflict pushes interpreters to seek independent solutions to address communication problems by inventing individual strategies to suit given situations. The wide range of strategies reported by the participants is creative and is found to be effective in addressing tricky cultural issues in interpreting. At the same time, the predominantly independent approaches to communication problems in interpreting represent a compromise which interpreters had to make within the monolingual environment of Australian hospitals. While inter-party collaboration is reported as desirable, the general attitude of HCPs to interpreting as a mechanistic activity makes it often untenable, pressuring interpreters to come up with their own strategies to address communication problems alone.

Finally, the findings highlight a striking resemblance between the past and the present in terms of interpreters' recommendations for HCPs. The similarity between the recommendations from the participants in this study and those from the first health care interpreters in the 1970s indicates that health care institutions need to pay attention to voices from interpreters and that more progress needs to be made in terms of institutional awareness of interpreting. This proves just how ignored interpreting continues to be, and confirms that its under-appreciation is a long-standing issue.

From a critical sociolinguistic perspective, the book is compelled by the evidence it has adduced to confirm that the under-appreciation of interpreting in Australia is intrinsically connected to monolingual ideologies operating at multiple levels. By paying attention to the hitherto-little-explored dimensions of linguistic, racial and class biases in health care interpreting, it highlights the under-appreciation of interpreting as a sociolinguistic problem which generates inequalities for other languages and their speakers. By bringing together interpreting and critical sociolinguistics, the book demonstrates the value of interdisciplinary approaches through which to expose minority struggles against dominant ideologies and practices. The demonstrated relations between interpreting and monolingualism are particularly useful for ongoing sociological and sociolinguistic approaches in the interpreting scholarship to explicate how societal attitudes to other languages and speakers impact the status of interpreting and interpreters. Conversely, examination of interpreters' status can also reveal societal relations with other languages and speakers, which suggests interpreting as a key site for further critical sociolinguistics investigations.

Taken together, the book highlights the urgent need to bring about changes to the ways in which interpreting is perceived and treated across various social and professional spaces. The next section discusses how to move forward.

7.2 Way forward

The findings of this book highlight the need to bridge the gap between the system, which is globally regarded as a model, and the actual level of awareness and practice relating to interpreting.

At the institutional level, the poor understanding of interpreting among HCPs can be addressed by mandating that HCPs be better trained in interpreting. Various states of Australia have guidelines on how to work with interpreters for health care practitioners (see NSW Health, 2017; Queensland Health, 2007; Victoria Department of Health and Human Services, 2017; Western Australia Department of Health, 2017 for example), yet the book shows that many HCPs significantly lack both understandings and abilities of how to work with interpreters. Interpreters in Australia are required to complete professional training to update their knowledge in relevant areas of work as part of requirements to renew their professional certifications (see National Accreditation Authority for Translators and Interpreters, n.d.). Corresponding efforts need to be made by HCPs too, by requiring them to take professional development training on the role of interpreting in health care work.

It is also important for universities to incorporate education and training on language barriers and interpreting. HCPs working in multicultural societies such as Australia are highly likely to encounter patients not fluent in the dominant language, and appropriate understanding of interpreting is critical to ensure successful communication. As far as can be learned, hardly any medical schools in Australia offer training in interpreting for students. If it began at university, students would be equipped with the necessary knowledge about how to work with interpreters. This will, in turn, help ensure quality of health care for patients from minority backgrounds. Without reciprocal responses from health care, the onus of addressing communication problems will continue to be placed on interpreters.

Furthermore, hospital systems need to change to accommodate the specific needs of interpreters and NESB patients. As discussed above (see Section 7.1.3; see also Section 5.4), interpreter-mediated consultations need to be given the sort of priority that ensures timely consultations to allow interpreters to work effectively and efficiently. It is also necessary to increase consultation time for interpreter-assisted communication to ensure full, quality communication for NESB patients. These small steps will certainly make a big difference in the health and quality of life of minority patients.

At the market level, it is urgent to improve the working conditions for interpreters, particularly payment. The recent pay increase for interpreters in the state of Victoria serves as a good example. After a static increase in interpreting wages for over 15 years, the Victorian government approved in 2018 a significant funding increase to improve the pay and working conditions of interpreters. The new plan included a 30 per cent increase in rates for standard face-to-face sessions and up to 48 per cent for telephone sessions, which marked the largest single funding boost for interpreter services in the state's history. The value of interpreting for social equity was clearly acknowledged in a statement released by the Ministry for Multicultural Affairs: "interpreters enable linguistically diverse communities to better access health, education and other critical services" (Estopace, 2018). Other states are encouraged to follow the suit of Victoria by recognising the critical roles which interpreters play in ensuring social inclusion of linguistic minorities.

The book also urges reviewing the ongoing market practice for hiring unqualified bilinguals for interpreting at a government level. People who appear to be fluent in languages may not understand complex medical terminology (Cheng et al., 2021) and non-professional interpreters for medical communications border on a health risk. Just like any professional, requirements for professional certification for interpreter recruitment need to be strictly followed. This is also important to boost the professional morale of interpreters. As discussed, acquiring interpreting certifications takes a significant amount of investment and effort and due professional recognition needs to be given to those who undergo them. It would require strengthening regulatory enforcement for language service providers to hire only qualified interpreters. It is also important to raise public awareness among clients about the importance of using certified interpreters by educating people about the risks of using non-professional interpreters.

At the societal level, it is important to raise public awareness of interpreting through which to make interpreting more visible. School education can play a key role in increasing awareness and understanding of interpreting and the related challenges encountered by migrants. Many people in Australia do not even know the difference between translation and interpreting (Cho, 2022). Many migrants in Australia struggle due to the lack of English language proficiency yet they are often blamed for not making enough effort to learn English. Negative views on language learning by migrants are the outcome of the monolingual mindset, which fails to understand the ties between skills in one language and those in other (Clyne, 2008).

Considering the social invisibility and under-appreciation of interpreting, it is encouraging to see the recent adoption of Auslan (Australian Sign Language) into Australian school curricula. In 2023, the New South Wales Government announced the introduction of Auslan as a second language in Australian primary and secondary schools from 2026. The formalisation of Auslan for curriculum inclusion represents a significant step towards diversity and inclusion, which is expected to improve public awareness of the importance of interpreting for deaf people (Australian Curriculum, n.d.). Teaching students about spoken interpreting and its importance for migrants is also expected to raise public awareness of migrant struggles, an understanding critical for strengthening social resilience.

Interpreting is generally considered invisible, yet the social invisibility of interpreting has rarely attracted attention. Being invisible is synonymous with being powerless. Being invisible also risks making minority voices unheard and problems unknown. As Bourdieu (1990) noted, it is important to notice power in places where it is least visible due to the invisible nature of power. Only through the problematising of what is taken for granted can a phenomenon become visible.

References

Australian Curriculum. (n.d.). *Introduction*. www.australiancurriculum.edu.au/f-10-curriculum/languages/auslan/introduction/

Bourdieu, P. (1990). *The logic of practice*. Polity Press.

Cheng, J. H., Wang, C., Jhaveri, V., Morrow, E., Li, S. T. T., & Rosenthal, J. L. (2021). Health care provider practices and perceptions during family-centered rounds with limited English-proficient families. *Academic Pediatrics*, *21*(7), 1223–1229. https://doi.org/10.1016/j.acap.2020.12.010

Cho, J. (2022). Hidden gems: Translators and interpreters in Australia play a critical if seldom seen role. *The Conversation*. https://theconversation.com/hidden-gems-translators-and-interpreters-in-australia-play-a-critical-if-seldom-seen-role-188603

Clyne, M. (2008). The monolingual mindset as an impediment to the development of plurilingual potential in Australia. *Sociolinguistic Studies*, *2*(3), 347–366. https://doi.org/10.1558/sols.v2i3.347

Clyne, M. G. (1991). *Community languages: The Australian experience*. Cambridge University Press.

Dam, H. V. (2017). Interpreter role, ethics and norms: Linking to professionalization. In M. Biagini, M. S. Boyd, & C. Monacelli (Eds.), *The changing role of the interpreter: Contextualising norms, ethics and quality standards* (pp. 228–239). Routledge.

D'Hayer, D. (2012). Public service interpreting and translation: Moving towards a (virtual) community of practice. *Meta*, *57*(1), 235–247. https://doi.org/10.7202/1012751ar

Eser, O., & Lai, M. (2018). Interview with Niki Baras, translators and interpreters Australia–A division of professionals Australia. *International Journal of Interpreter Education*, *10*(2), 73–78.

Estopace, E. (2018, July 18). Major pay increase marks big win for interpreters in Australian state of Victoria. *Slator*.

Hage, G. (2012). *White nation: Fantasies of white supremacy in a multicultural society*. Routledge.

Hale, S. B., & Napier, J. (2016). "We're just kind of there": Working conditions and perceptions of appreciation and status in court interpreting. *Target*, *28*(3), 351–371. https://doi.org/10.1075/target.28.3.01hal

Hearn, J. M. (1981). *The unrecognised professionals*. Education Research and Development Committee.

Hlavac, J. (2015). Formalizing community interpreting standards: A cross-national comparison of testing systems, certification conventions and recent ISO guidelines. *International Journal of Interpreter Education*, *7*(2), 21–38.

Mikkelson, H. (1996). The professionalization of community interpreting. In M. O'Keeffe (Ed.), *Global vision: Proceedings of the 37th annual conference of the american translators association* (pp. 77–89). American Translators Association.

National Accreditation Authority for Translators and Interpreters. (n.d.). *Recertification*. www.naati.com.au/certification/recertification/

NSW Health. (2017). *Standard Procedures for Working with Health Care Interpreters*. www1.health.nsw.gov.au/pds/ActivePDSDocuments/PD2017_044.pdf

Queensland Health. (2007). *Working with Interpreters: Guidelines*. www.health.qld.gov.au/__data/assets/pdf_file/0033/155994/guidelines_int.pdf

Rodriguez-Losada, D. (2019). Working conditions as a translator/interpreter in Australia: A personal overview. In A. Armando, I. Öztürk, & D. Aliu (Eds.), *Conceiving migration and communication in a global perspective* (pp. 21–29). Cambridge Scholars Publishing.

Victoria Department of Health and Human Services. (2017). *Language Services Policy*. www.dhhs.vic.gov.au/publications/language-services-policy-and-guidelines

Western Australia Department of Health. (2017). *WA Health System Language Services Policy Guidelines*. https://ww2.health.wa.gov.au/~/media/Files/Corporate/Policy%20Frameworks/Communications/Policy/WA%20Health%20System%20Language%20Services%20Policy/Supporting/WA-Health-System-Language-Services-Policy-Guidelines.pdf

Index

Note: Tables are indicated by **bold**.

FSC
www.fsc.org
MIX
Papier | Fördert gute Waldnutzung
FSC® C083411

Kolibri 360 GmbH
Ferdinand-Jühlke-Straße 7
99095 Erfurt, Deutschland
produktsicherheit@kolibri360.de